With great thanks to Ian Belcher for his
invaluable editorial input and energetic
refreshment of this story.

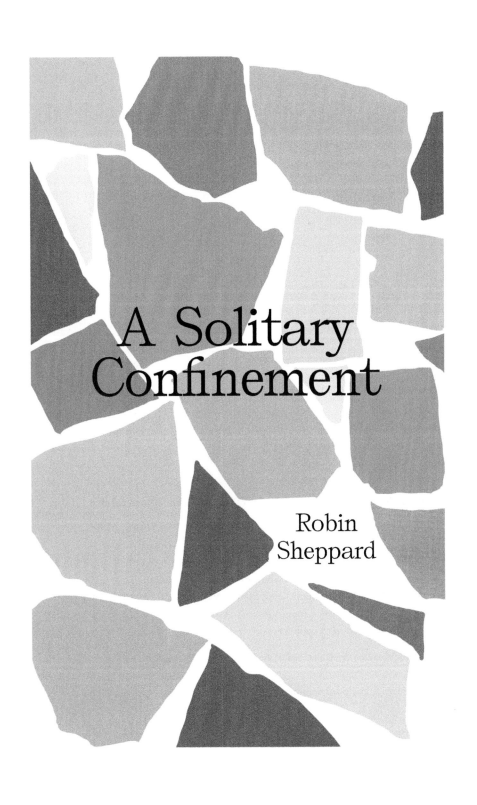

A Solitary Confinement

Robin Sheppard

A Solitary Confinement

First published in 2007
Second Edition published in 2019 by
Panoma Press Ltd
48 St Vincent Drive, St Albans, Herts, AL1 5SJ UK
info@panomapress.com
www.panomapress.com

Cover design by Charlie Sheppard
Typeset by Karen Gladwell

ISBN 978-1-784521-21-9

This book is available online and in all good bookstores.

Printed and bound in Great Britain by TJ International Ltd, Padstow, Cornwall

Preface

A decade after *A Solitary Confinement*, Robin Sheppard's remarkable, moving and darkly humorous account of fighting back against the ravages of Guillain-Barré syndrome – written without use of notes or hands – he revisits the debilitating, often bewildering experience. This revised version adds flesh to the bones, updating his story with a look at the legacy of a terrible illness, while catching up with some of the main players who graced the original drama.

Dedication

To G and B and SMRC

Contents

1

Fall and Decline

A Solitary Confinement

CHAPTER ONE

Fall and Decline

I t's one of those cold, breath-condensing, sombre days: the type with no other purpose than to prelude Christmas. Local shops are running out of mincemeat and brandy, the scrawniest fir trees being dragged along pavements by even scrawnier children and conversation is dominated by charity bucket holders exhorting passers-by to "give generously".

The lack of late afternoon daylight casts a jet black curtain across the street as I carry my clementine- and walnut-laden shopping bag up the pathway to the front door, peering at the candles flickering in the front window. The tree is up and cards hung: a view to make Scrooge weep.

Yet all is not well. It's 19th December and I've started to experience stabs of pain in my back. Pins and needles have begun to affect my senses, I'm losing feeling in my stomach and my arms and legs are heavy. I have a dry cough and am seriously tired. The flu must be coming.

The following day blurs as I notice a remarkably rapid reduction in my powers of alliteration and motor function. A sense of agony is erupting from my spine, intensifying and leaking across my body. Ordinary everyday tasks – blowing my nose or picking up a telephone – require monumental effort.

Reflexes are slowing, normal sensations draining away. Driving down the motorway in the early evening takes great concentration and several stops. Staying in the correct lane is a challenge in itself, so I slow down to mask my erratic steering. Add in a hacking cough and drowsiness and this promises to be the mother of all colds.

When I reach my destination, in the spa town of Bath, I'm sweating. I struggle out of the car and my walking is uneven and hesitant. I don't feel safe to drive again but, of course, ignore my own sage advice and head off to a nearby office next morning. My working doesn't last long. The room seems to be spinning, I keep keeling over like a drunken sailor. I even miss the first coffee break – it must be bad. There's no option but to cancel my appointments and go back to bed. Somehow the car gets me there.

I'm staying upstairs in my father's house, from where I try to ring my GP. After six abortive attempts I manage to get through and describe my conditions. It's apparently insufficient to merit a home visit. So, placebos all round. He prescribes painkillers. The iceberg has struck the transatlantic liner and his emergency procedures dictate a brisk shuffle of the deckchairs.

It might appear to an overburdened family doctor that I have a heavyweight cold but paracetamol will most definitely not suffice. My breathing is becoming irregular, I feel intermittently faint and then quite lucid. By mid-afternoon I can no longer walk. Somehow I get out of bed, grimly determined to get to the loo. I fall across the dressing table, steady myself and head for the door.

I get as far as the the landing, little realising these are to be my last steps for a very long time. Rather like Mutley from the classic *Wacky Races* cartoons, I have run over the edge of the cliff and, although my legs still spin round, there's no longer any ground below me. At this highest point of suspended animation all is still and serene. Shep, I think to myself, you're in big trouble.

I crash to the ground face upwards and there I stay… and stay. And I'm still desperate to pee. Help is needed. Stark naked, save for a nearby Nokia 3210 to spare my blushes, I try to send an SOS on my mobile phone. The first flurry of texts emanate from my fingertips before they give up the struggle, forcing my knuckles to take over. I'm at a loss, not knowing how to describe my malaise without spreading untold panic. I can't speak to anyone because I can't lift the phone towards my mouth. Gravity is in overdrive. Indeed I'm only managing to expedite the texts by resting the phone on my hip and tipping my head to one side to see what I'm doing.

It's a truly dreadful and terrifying passage of time. A period when the minutes stand still. I despatch a clarion cry for assistance but it's overtaken by the predictive text machinery. The simple expression 'Help I am in trouble can't move' turns into a very illuminating 'Gely h an go trotter abou note'. Little wonder people ignore me.

Remembering my father's deafness I cry out at the top of my voice. Dad, bless him, is downstairs watching *Countdown* and busy choosing between his vowels and his consonants with the television on full volume. Carol Vorderman stands between me and salvation. Will I ever forgive her for this trespass, or that rubber dress?

I try to move. Nothing happens. I'm completely and utterly immobile. After what seems like eternity there's a knock at the front door. Fortunately, avuncular Albert, our Irish neighbour, has come round to drop off some sausages, as you do. Albert hears my cries straight away and, as he climbs the stairs, comforts me. "Jesus, look at the state of you. Have you been on the falling down juice?"

I apologise for my nakedness while ever genial Albert takes control and calls for an ambulance. Somehow he gets me into a pair of bright lemon pyjamas, puts a £10 note and mobile phone into my breast pocket and exclaims, "That'll 'see you right'."

CHAPTER TWO

Fall and Decline

The ambulance drivers are solicitous in the extreme, placing me on to a stretcher which converts into a chair. Three people lift me downstairs whilst giving me regular bursts of oxygen. Something's clearly wrong, but what? It's 21st December, I'm about to be trussed up like a turkey in the Accident and Emergency unit of Bath's Royal United Hospital. How can the shortest day of the year feel so long?

So determined am I to hold on to my breathing, I can't rest, petrified that if I fall asleep I'll never wake. My voice is rapidly weakening as the balance between talking and inhaling air grows more tenuous. There's so much I want to say, endless questions formulating but which will be left unasked. Each word and sentence seems to reduce my lung capacity. This is the real fight. If I can just push back against this paralysing rape of my neck, chest, throat and tongue. "To have and to hold," I keep repeating. "To have and to hold."

The battle rages for hours. The war will run into days. My captor is gathering strength like a hurricane muscling up in the mid-Atlantic, its advance gusts clearing any sign of resistance until it's ready for the final full-force assault on my constitution.

The senior consultant, who patrols the Accident and Emergency department like an officious sergeant major, doesn't tell me what he thinks my illness might be. He merely explains that my breathing will probably give out soon and I shouldn't be surprised or alarmed. Easier said than done. I'm quite attached to my breathing and have no intention of letting go of this much practised skill.

Various appliances have been rigged up around me to help stabilise my condition. The usual suspects, lined up in an identity parade beside my bed, including a saline drip, blood extraction piping and an applicator to ply me with painkillers, are the only items I can identify. The faces of the staff, other patients and layout of the room barely register. These days leading up to Christmas are stolen from me. Time seems to stand still. Some greater power presses the pause button and erases nearly three days.

I'm inundated with the first wave of nearest and dearest who are struggling to come to terms with what appears to have happened to me. I want to reassure them, to show I'm remaining upbeat despite my body confirming the severity of the condition. They look really concerned. Whether they want to provide this damning endorsement or not, the choice has been removed. No one who comes to see me at this time can hide the terror that my countenance induces.

Breathing is getting shallower and more difficult by the hour, then by the minute. I want to fight, to keep pushing out the old air and gulping down the new. I slide in what air I can while an alien force has slipped behind my tongue to shunt the oxygen out faster, then faster still. I can barely talk now. No surrender… I will… fight this. Batten down the hatches. There's a storm a comin' in.

Here comes that moment when you're supposed to see all of your past life before you. Yes, here it comes… can't breathe, can't speak… pressure on my lungs, Jesus, Mary… no air, I'm drowning here. Help me, sweet Joseph, can you answer this prayer? I'm gulping, gasping… distended lips mouthing like a freshly caught trout, eyes rolling in their sockets. I can't breathe, I can't breeeee… falling, falling, falling… all… the way… down.

It's Christmas Eve. Staff are running towards me in slow motion, the lights going on and off, there is an overwhelming white noise. Finally my breathing collapses as though I'm just dropping off to sleep and a sudden sense of falling takes me away. I want to shout "Don't fret, it's only a myoclonic jerk… happens all the time." But all is rushing. Trees ripped out of the sodden earth are flying past my window, branches flaying. I'm leaving… cheerio… ta-ta … goodnight.

I pass out…

Life, real honest-to-goodness life, with its catastrophes, murders and out-of-the-blue inheritances of inconceivable wealth, happens almost inevitably in newspapers. Surely life is not happening to me. Not now. Not here. Not with so much still to do, so many songs to sing, operas to write and words to say.

I don't want to be dead. But I just have… died, I think. Yet if I'm actually thinking, a sentient being, I can't have. So where and what am I now?

I open my eyes. Listen. Smell. There must be clues. I can't find any. I want to but… still… can't. All is surreal. I'm drifting like tumbleweed down a deserted midwest street. Out of control, captured by capricious winds, rolling over then around and up and beyond misplaced boulders. Now I'm falling again, drifting away to different vistas.

Images, cloudy and opaque, flash in front as if drawn from the deepest fevered vortex. There are stiff white sheets and pale green walls, dark blue uniforms and powerful extraction fans high in the ceiling. Strip lights in curious reflective housing appear as works of art beneath a roof of endless rectangular off-white panels, while reflective silver material is warped and bent like funfair mirrors.

Twist my head a fraction to the left and there's a bridge, seaside and wooden beach groins. Turn it a tad to the right and the lights mutate into reflections of motor cars reversing by a hundred kerbs: a constantly distorting kaleidoscopic view created by each millimetric shift of my eyeball as I look upwards in search of reassurance.

I stare at the ceiling with an unblinking gaze, unable to see my feet or the scratches on my hands and arms where tubes have been inserted. Something is not right about my neck. I don't think it belongs to me. Nor can I see or sense my fingertips or toes. My back appears to be broken in two. I can't lift my head off the pillow or, indeed, move any part of my body save my mouth which can open and shut like a ventriloquist's dummy yet produces no sound.

So is this heaven or hell? Which one did the good Lord choose? Does it really matter, anyway? I feel so abused and abased, so battered and bashed, so comprehensively crushed.

Or maybe it's neither. Maybe I'm still alive. Maybe the doctors managed to rescue me from the typhoon and, just maybe, someone has looked so kindly on me that there's a second coming. It's a new beginning, a second half, a chance for redemption. Perhaps my life can start again with alternative rules and a whole fresh agenda.

It is, after all, Christmas Day, I think. How auspicious. How prescient. What a day to be born again. How finely balanced is that glass by which we judge whether life is half-full or half-empty. Just being alive should provide all the knowledge we need. My glass will always be deemed half-full from now on. The time will come to fight back but at this moment I need assistance – and lots of it.

Help is indeed at hand, but what fanfare will usher it in? Something majestic, even priapic, to mark this reprieve would be sweet, perhaps a little Beethoven girding our loins with *Ode to Joy* at full volume? What will it be?

- CHAPTER THREE -

Fall and Decline

My reawakening does not receive the classical masterpiece I believe it deserves. The distant strains of Noddy Holder exhorting "So here it is, Merry Christmas, everybody's having fun" mingle with the scent of mulled wine and mince pies wafting around the unfamiliar ward. Where am I? Is this the intensive care unit? Nurses appear wearing red antlers and tinsel, blissfully unaware I have a demon scratching the tip of my nose and am powerless to do anything about it.

And so begins the next chapter of life. Without warning my torso has been taken hostage. I haven't given permission for this to happen, nor was I expecting it, but there's no doubt I'm facing a second half.

I'm now trapped in my own body. This is a very different form of imprisonment with the cell in the head and the exercise yard closed. Still, it could be worse. There aren't any cockroaches or bars on the windows. In time maybe I can start to plan the escape from Alcatraz, but not today. I clearly have work to do first. For a start I have to stay alive. The autopilot controlling my destiny has been reprogrammed with just one target: descend with alacrity towards the inexorable crash landing.

Any sense of day and night has disappeared. The only way I can tell which is which is by studying the faces looking after me, as some people only work nights. The evening should herald a quiet period but in intensive care there's no peace for the wicked or the unwell at any time. With other senses receding my ears are in overdrive. Noise is my latest assailant, twisting and tormenting me. The 27 people on the ward all need immediate help, and each is attached to several devices which activate a sound when supplies run out or there's a change in behaviour. It sounds like an orchestra permanently tuning up. Whiz, bang, crash, wallop, plonk, kerpow... and there's no sign of a conductor to bring them to heel.

Surely intensive care is somewhere you go when you're really, really ill? I don't belong here, I'll be as right as rain soon enough. There's some perfectly logical explanation for this minor inconvenience. This is such an alien experience. Perhaps I've been placed in this penitentiary to study absolution.

I can't grasp the layout of the ward, images are too vague and transitory to cement in the brain. But I can still count, and they move me seven times from one bed to another as each successive more urgent case is admitted. Now I understand how those old-fashioned filing systems were supposed to work. I'm fulfilling the role of the lonely memo which required attention when it first came in but which matters less and less against the daily influx of new crises.

Interruptions become a new way of life. Change is constant and the only staple part of the staff's diet is adrenaline. So challenging are some of the cases that they devour every ounce of the doctors' and nurses' concentration.

Each new arrival takes precedence, drama upon drama. None are well enough to form any alliance or kinship with, and their relations are too concerned with their own nightmares. It's a very singular time.

Just when I think things are starting to stabilise, another of my faculties closes down. Happiness has gone into hiding, hopefully just around the corner, temporarily out of sight and mind. It leaves a vacuum which fills with trepidation and bursts of unbounded misery.

In such despair impressions, half-formed, come with links that might just catch hold of each other. By happenstance, or serendipity, I might generate some modest coalescence but I don't know what to fasten on to, so emasculating and hostile are my darkest moments.

Like most men I've left Christmas shopping to the last minute. Yes I've wrapped some gifts for loved ones, but while the Sellotape, scissors and wrapping paper, along with the frankincense and myrrh, are all under the same roof, they're no use to anyone without assembly. Worrying about Christmas presents is akin to the irrational fear of suffering an accident without fresh underpants. Yet in this place of acute vulnerability, where life is trying to dodge death by holding on to a gossamer-thin thread, such trivia starts to dominate.

It's a curious place to be in this state of debilitation. The mind appears to be untouched, the body clearly isn't. In fact, it seems to be determined to move as far away from my brain as possible, leaving a point about halfway up my neck and above relatively intact. Like a macabre cartoon, I imagine my brain alone in a pickling jar with pipes leading into various components of my body which lie strewn around a laboratory. My liver bubbles away in a test tube, my thighs simmer in cider flagons, and my arms are in a Belfast sink: a horribly fragmented jigsaw puzzle. Messages from my brain to my limbs bounce back like unwanted emails. Where has my body gone? It still appears to be there, yet the disconnect is so profound that a new reality has to be accepted. And quickly. I wonder if surfer dudes off Hawaii feel this kind of in-body out-of-body experience as they catch the perfect wave and enter its green room to snake, pirouette and arc towards the shore. Mine is an altogether drier experience, particularly as I'm now under a regime of nil by mouth and the closest I get to water is having an ice cube rubbed around my lips. It has become fearfully thirsty in the Sahara of my brain.

Unable to move or speak, communication is impossible save for the messages transmitted by my appearance – and I can't even control that. There are several tubes around me, two of which I watch being pushed into my left nostril. Designed to take over the work of my failing stomach, they add a certain elegance to my outfit, the colours complementing my, by now, peppermint pyjamas.

The first tube measures a meagre 40cm but warrants a senior doctor and three auxiliaries to rotate and steer the invader through my nose, down the throat and into the stomach to siphon off excess air. The second, a more impressive 60cm, takes far more twisting by two sets of hands to turn the tip beyond the tummy into food absorption headquarters.

The doctor maintains a dull running commentary throughout, with all the inflection of an automated Speak Your Weight machine. I, however, imagine an excitable Murray Walker leading the description 'as into the hairpin bends races the tube before executing a perfect overtaking manoeuvre through the chicanes, on the way to the duodenum'.

A hole has been cut into the lowest point of my neck to receive the most important pipe. It supplies air into my lungs, which rise and fall at a regular pace. I'm also plumbed into a life-support machine. It's intrusive, scratchy, overwhelming and ever so welcome. Without it, if I'd been born in another country or previous generation, I'd be dead. With it I have a chance.

My thoughts wander from crystal clarity to depths of despondence, fug and confusion. I come to rely upon the steady rhythm of my controlled breathing, not just for my obvious physical need but as the tempo for my mental mantras, repeated over and over, "Fight. Fight. Fight." The beat is steadier than Ringo Starr, and almost as monotonous as one of his drum solos.

The external manifestation of this illness is my immobile limbs and trunk. But the internal machinations are more mysterious. The eyelids gum together reducing or curtailing visibility, so that seeing clearly is an event separated by days and only lasting minutes. My mouth dries to such an extent that I need fake saliva to be sprayed under my tongue.

My bottom is on strike too. Useful if you don't have the right change for the station loo in Zagreb on a freezing night, but hopeless if it lasts for weeks. Feeling through the hands – other than constant pain – has disappeared, as has awareness of any internal sensation. Hot or cold water on my flesh feels the same as a rough towel. It seems a magnetic force has wrapped itself around me and is repelling all comers. Yet I crave movement. Any nurse prepared to help me move on my side, rearrange pillows or adjust my various pipes becomes an instant candidate for beatification. I watch them act out their parts in the hospital play through one or the other half-open eyelid.

Giving care on a one-to-one basis to critically ill people is quite a vocation. I'm sure I wouldn't have the dedication, steely resolve and altruism it requires. But boy, do they impress. The staff come from all walks of life, from Spain, the Philippines, Kenya, even Bristol. Some have been born in the road next to the hospital and never left the county, much less been abroad. Yet all are bound by one shared instinct: to do their utmost to keep their charges in the best condition possible.

On an especially harrowing night I overhear the death of a mother who has endured operation after operation. As I can't turn my head to see the characters perform, it's like listening to a ghastly radio play. The family are dysfunctional in the extreme, and the young daughter clearly has no love for her stepfather. To hear the cries of that poor seven-year-old go on and on as she realises her mother has died is excruciating. No one, least of all those close to her, can provide comfort or succour. What a chilling welcome to *Cold Comfort Farm*.

CHAPTER FOUR

Fall and Decline

A *human being experiences himself, his thoughts and feelings as something separated from the rest, a kind of optical delusion of his consciousness. This delusion is a kind of prison for us, restricting us to our personal desires and to affection for a few persons nearest us. Our task must be to free ourselves from this prison by widening our circle of compassion to embrace all living creatures and the whole of nature in its beauty.*"

Out of my mouth such words might appear pious nonsense but they're actually the observation of someone with a slightly bigger brain, a certain Mr Albert Einstein (although I can't help but note his odd use of the word *optical*). Now Albert undoubtedly had a point – he usually did – but I hope you'll forgive me if, in my straitened circumstances, I disregard the greater good of all living creatures and stay in my 'prison' for just a little while longer. I'd like to flashback in time and take you on a short, gentle stroll through my existence so far: my personal and family life, as well as my career.

I've never heard of Guillain-Barré, let alone encountered it, up until this moment. It's fair to say that I've been blessed in many ways. In fact life has been pretty sunny from the get-go. Quite literally. I was born into the Mediterranean heat and cloudless cyan skies of Malta, with the honey-hued stone of its vibrant, colourful harbour etched into my memory. My family's return to Britain when I was three years old might have been a poor transfer on the weather front – although my first exposure to February West Country drizzle perhaps forged some iron in my soul – but I can't complain. The move paved the way for a gloriously happy upbringing in the Georgian splendour of Bath. Friendships were formed in school that have lasted and deepened over the decades. True mates indeed.

Through it all my parents were a wonderful guiding influence and my father, now knocking on towards 90, remains a huge presence, anchor and strength in my life. As I hit my own half-century, I find I'm now the proud father of two sons in their late teens, Sam the elder (the musical one) and Charlie (the artistic one). While my marriage ended, I remain good friends with their mother and my first wife Georgina, known always as George. I'm now partnered and supported quite brilliantly by the effervescent and indomitable Suzanne, known by all as Suzi.

As for my career, well, it has been an unfettered existence working in places that bear little resemblance to the usual definition of a factory or office. It was a universe that largely revolved around five-star hotels, most cocooned in manicured gardens with fine wines, fabulous *foie gras* and outrageous flower arrangements. All the establishments were speckled with well-heeled customers enjoying an environment in which the anticipation of their needs was paramount. Whatever Sir or Madam wanted – unless it was totally outrageous – they tended to get.

I served my time, of course. Having started as an enthusiastic junior on the lower rungs of the business, I'd quickly learned the ropes and risen up the ranks, gaining vital experience en route, emerging as a hotelier who delighted in operating – and sometimes opening – many of the very best British hotels. We're talking about the likes of Bodysgallen Hall in North Wales, an extraordinary manor house swaddled in luxuriant woods, built over a period of 600 years with a five-storey, 13th century watch house at its historic heart. Several of the properties picked up gongs for 'hotel of the year' – successes that helped lay the foundation for a specialist hotel management group I started with a few like-minded chums.

As once with Rome, all roads in Britain appeared to lead to London. Once there I presided over an empire of a dozen or so glamorous hotels, beloved of international guests, celebrities and paparazzi. These were capital gems featuring listed architecture of the Grade 1 variety, decadent décor and period fixtures, along with gourmet cuisine regularly adorned with Michelin stars and AA rosettes. Add in some parkland surroundings worthy of Capability Brown and it would be fair to say this was an untroubled workplace.

It wasn't all hotels, mind you. Taking time out along the way I founded the Ty-Nant mineral water company with its iconic, deep blue, skittle-shaped bottles, followed by a niche, adult, soft drinks business whose exotic natural blends are stocked by the likes of Pret A Manger. In so doing I accidentally became a successful entrepreneur as well as a role model for many a novice hotel student.

As I said, a lucky man. A very lucky man. There was nothing, not even the extreme pedantry of privileged five-star guests – an entirely different version of intensive care – that had prepared me for an enforced claustrophobic stay in a communal room with antiseptic wipes rather than sweet-scented Balmain toiletries. At this moment the past isn't just a foreign country, it's a different universe.

CHAPTER FIVE

Fall and Decline

"What's Guillain-Barré syndrome?" I want to say to the young doctor who has just broken the news. But my expression will have to suffice. Perhaps unsurprisingly she has become good at reading eyes. Very good.

Trying to be concise she lists what she knows about the illness. To summarise…

It affects more than 1,000 people a year in the UK.

The immune system gets the wrong message, thinks it's under attack and so attacks itself.

Most patients recover within two years… but for some it takes up to seven.

It's a slow and exhausting process and you'll always be left with residual tiredness.

I'm sure she tells me many more things, but I'm stuck at the mention of two years… this seems a long time. A very long time indeed. How can I put this into context? Pain, tears, happiness, joy, laughter and loss were all colours in the past rainbow of experience. Do I have any reserves in latent suspension waiting to be activated? How do you remove such a vast level of faculty without replacing it with something? Surely there's a way I can cope with this new reality by gaining strength from previous challenges. Inject industrial quantities of self-belief perhaps? Or maybe now is the time to really understand the family motto *Dum Spiro Spero* (While I Breathe I Hope).

Hope was also my mother's middle name and surely everything comes if man will only wait. So is waiting for hope to show up to be my new hobby? No. Let's be practical here. Let's start with the foundations and build up. Normative needs sit at the bottom of the hierarchy of needs, way below fancy cars and fine holidays, and even further below the state of self-actualisation that we're all supposedly searching for. But when you're thrown so wildly off course from the usual aspirations of a selfish life, normative needs become the only focus. How you breathe, eat and sleep is so important you're incapable of thinking of anything, let alone anyone, else.

And then there's the fear of the unknown. It causes us to be afraid of many things from death to public speaking – absurdly claimed to rank the higher of the two – and being buried alive is apparently the most reviled way to die. According to Edgar Allen Poe it is "beyond question, the most terrifying of those extremes which has ever fallen to the lot of mere mortals". This is no apocryphal moment for me. Yes, fate has determined to bury me inside my own custom-built coffin. I can't detect six feet of earth on top of my chest perhaps, yet the effect on my ability to move from this amorphous state is identical.

I'm desperate to fight back, to break out of this singular cell. My anguish and gut-wrenching melancholy are palpable. But there has to be a way out. I'd best form my own escape committee. I don't just need people around me to do good deeds, offer prayers and roll their rosaries – or a gospel choir to extol the virtues of born-again religion – I need resonance by the bucketload. The main problem is that the chief supplier of this season's deluxe, must-have, special offer resonance is out of town. I'm in charge.

Everybody close to me wants to be useful and indeed they are, in their own way, as helpful as you'd expect them to be. That is all anyone looking in on the internee can do though. Unless I take charge, setting my own pace and agenda, the building blocks will never be put in the right order. This may sound ungracious or vain; it's neither. It's just what life does when one person's destiny is knocked so far out of line that there's a tangible distance between you and other people. Those closest still seem adjacent, but they aren't in the house with me anymore, they're outside looking in. Concern is etched on their every facial expression. My new role is to be the object of this concern. I've been absented from smelling the roses in the garden, and no amount of protestation will let me outdoors again. You can feel the presence of your nearest and dearest, their scent, their warmth and their passion. It just doesn't taste the same: too many of your six senses have been removed or terminated.

The sense of helplessness is all-engulfing. Apart from being able to move my head from side to side and open and close my mouth (and occasionally my gummed-up eyes) there is no other movement I can initiate or sound I can make. Why should anyone want to talk to me? I can't open up a discussion, voice approval, stimulate debate or tell a witty tale.

Yet the nurses' most restorative medicine is the one-way conversations they hold with me. They proceed around the ward in gangs of two or three, checking vital supplies are getting through: intravenous drips for the water, immunoglobulin to repair damaged nerve endings, and food through the nose, while painkillers arrive by syringe, spit by spray, and depression suppression by crushed tablet. They fluff up my bed, straighten my sheets, mop my brow and they talk to me. Several are skilled in the execution of all these tasks but many fail with the last.

Dignity is not something I've ever considered becoming compromised. Sure enough though, it has disappeared in record time. The inability to control bodily functions is hardly a shock to those who live and work in hospitals, but for people like me, new to the game, it's something you can't stop wanting to apologise for. I'm sorry you have to wash my armpits, fit me with a catheter, replace my soiled trousers and apply eye drops to prevent the lids from gluing together. If I could only talk I'd tell you how grateful I am.

It really doesn't matter. You've entered a new universe in which the old rules no longer apply. No one cares about the sensibilities, vexations or inappropriate behaviour. Making a mess of the bedclothes is absolutely the done thing, it's appropriate and apposite. Discard at a stroke 50 years of prejudicial learning about what's right and what's wrong. Forget what constitutes dignified behaviour, and don't spare the horses.

This metamorphosis is quite a leap of faith, yet so inevitable you simply shouldn't waste time searching for an alternative. Whatever my dignity used to be no longer is. It is an ex-dignity, it is deceased. Like many a parrot before it, my dignity has fallen off its perch. Fear has outmanoeuvred dignity. It is now all-pervading, mainly of the unknown but particularly a fear of likelihood and statistics.

A more senior doctor arrives proffering research from Japan and Denmark. She explains she is pleased I do not appear to have contracted polio – a fright

29

in itself – but the statistics in her research garnered from *The Lancet* make her believe I'm unlikely to walk again. This information is unwelcome and unfeeling. You could knock me down with a feather, if I wasn't lying flat on my back anyway. You can try tickling me with it too, but you won't get very far. I'm suddenly in the most bellicose mood.

You see, there are two types of Guillain-Barré, and in true fast-food style I have decided to 'go large'. This means I have the axonal variety of the syndrome, which damages the nerve endings more thoroughly than its less capricious sister. The myelin which protects the nerves – a bit like the grey plastic insulation around copper wiring – is stripped away more vigorously, leaving exposed nerves to short-circuit each other. Apparently I'm an unusual case because of the pace of the decline. It's more common for people to worsen over two to three weeks. I've gone under in days. Furthermore the syndrome usually attacks only part of your body, say from the waist down. It very rarely strikes so completely and at such velocity.

What exactly do you say to a doctor who has just delivered the news you're unlikely to walk again? Well I take the hostile route and in the faintest whisper hiss back, "I most certainly will walk again." I'm cross. I've lost the diplomacy to be polite.

The anger coursing through my veins is a good thing. It tells me I have the will to fight, and that I'm not going to give in to this illness. I'm absolutely determined to make as full a recovery as possible. I kid myself my message has been received, but the rant remains private. No one can understand a word I'm trying to say.

The assured, urbane doctor continues to enlighten me. There is more demising to do. Things are not bad enough yet. Apparently the 16 days following the collapse of one's breathing will see the worst of the attack on the nervous system. There is a period thereafter when the deterioration bottoms out, before you begin the ascent from the foothills of Kilimanjaro to the top of the peak, as slowly as any novice mountaineer without sherpa, road map or woolly socks. At least the oxygen supply problem will be the reverse of that experienced by mountaineers. As I recover, my ability to consume and process air will improve.

- CHAPTER SIX -
Fall and Decline

In cricketing parlance I've taken a hit for six. Mentally I'm all over the shop. My inner family sanctum have put their lives on hold. I've ruined their Christmas as well as my own. My indefatigable partner Suzi has abandoned her family festivities and made a beeline for my bedside. And there she stays, offering pragmatic, unfailingly cheerful and very firm support. Without her devotion I'd be an emotional cripple, with it I'm just a wreck.

The effect on my family is, in a way, more difficult to cope with than the effect on myself. Watching my elder teenage son Sam recoil in horror at his first sight of me lying prostrate, unable to articulate the shock as if he has just witnessed a horrendous train derailment, is hard. George, my first wife, and Charlie my younger son, bless them, are desperately trying to work out what practical help will make life more tolerable for me, and remove pressure behind the scenes by taking care of my 89-year-old father. Dad isn't strong enough to go out shopping for himself and his own health is in such a parlous state that my malaise is bound to have the wrong effect.

Suzi's two adult children, Charles and Amanda, come down from London with their best friend James. They burst into tears straight away. Mark you, I do look especially ill today as my complexion has turned a funereal shade of grey. I want to cry too, but tears inside will have to suffice. Grandpa Charles, Uncle Tom and Dickie Blo are also wonderfully constant in their affections, taking more than their fair share of visiting duties and assisting behind the scenes.

Another day, another friend, one enjoying the identical spelling of my name, Robin Sheppard, visits the ward. Armed with photographic libraries, including holiday snapshots – trips to the Arabian Gulf and wild nights of excess in Paris – and, most spectacularly, the new fence around his son's postage stamp front lawn, he drones on and on. I'm usually happier if creosote is applied to the timber before construction and, indeed, might have ventured this opinion in a less life-threatening environment. Clearly, Robin has absolutely no understanding of what's needed by a seriously ill person at such a critical point. The words intensive care haven't provided a single clue and his well-intentioned but misguided behaviour is so out of kilter I'm unable to cope.

This visit is particularly instructive. It teaches me that I want people to visit but am incapable of concentrating for more than ten minutes at a time. Or five if fences are on the agenda. Some might say I've never been tolerant of people when I'm not feeling sociable but my yawning, and closing of one eye or the other, bring my boorishness to new heights. Pleasantries and good manners have their place for sure, but right now they've been evacuated to a safe house, for their protection.

Food in the intensive care department is something I can only picture. All sensory delights are denied, no awareness of seasoning, flavour or texture is available. Meals are a sickly green, soup-like mixture from a syringe, injected into the tube in my nose to bypass the stomach straight into the duodenum. The stomach has only agreed to air removal, not consumption during its sabbatical. Other patients are fed in a similar fashion. Red mullet mousseline with tomato coulis, accompanied by a crisp dry Sauvignon to enhance the piquancy, does not feature.

When you're really ill it's most likely you'll die from pneumonia in the early onset rather than the disease for which you were first admitted to hospital. This entitles an army of physio terrorists to appear at your bedside at will, moving with the stealth of the Spanish Inquisition. Without warning, just as you feel you've come to terms with the discrepancies in your breathing from excess mucus, one of these ferocious girls clambers across your chest, opens the flap in your neck and attaches what feels like the middle bit of a bagpipe to the hole where your tracheotomy was. In one deft movement, she turns you on your side, shakes you vigorously and squeezes the bagpipe in and out whilst explaining, "That's a good bit of gunk gurgling away on your chest, cough for me now, that's it, go on, one more!"

These interruptions punctuate my day five or six times. Otherwise I'm half-awake and half-asleep, drifting randomly from night to day. I imagine some murky lagoon under low mist where I stay afloat, bobbing up and down like flotsam, shipping too much water and struggling for air. The analgesics mask reality behind a façade of hallucination and detachment.

I have now been in hospital for almost three weeks. There may be a sharply defined world out there but I can't see it, existing in a semi-conscious arcadian dream where all faces are silhouettes, all noises muffled, all colours smudged. Indeterminate voices whisper nonsense as spectres and ghouls make merry with my heart. It is a desolate wasteland in the mind when the palliatives erase your concentration, cutting you loose from your moorings to drift through colours and clouds, vapours, eddies and whirlpools. In a rare moment of clarity I picture a man arriving at the Voluntary Euthanasia Superstore to keep the appointment with his maker. After being shown to his room, he's asked his favourite colour so they can set the shade over his bed before he's posed the question everyone should have an answer ready for: "What kind of music would you like to die to?"

I know. Do you?

Later that day a kindly nurse tells me she knows how to help me hear my own voice. At a time when I can't talk at all this seems very strange. Rather like using a key to peel back the lid on a sardine tin, she curls back the flap in my neck, tweaks my vocal chords with a blade and invites me to speak. Something comes out, similar to the squeak clowns emit when they swallow helium from a balloon. That's the good news.

The bad news is the smell. I suddenly smell death. It is acrid yet sweet, centuries-old but so vivid and current. The blend of dryness and dust from old parchment, blown up my nostrils by the devil himself, startles me. It had seemed such a kind and considerate suggestion by the nurse, yet here I am, truly scared. Not only do I think I've seen the other side, but I'm now smelling it too. I can hear Albinoni's *Adagio* accompanying the movement of my ashes. I feel icy cold. Death is dancing on my tongue, a jig of delight perhaps, mocking my many human failings. The image is chilling in its sharpness… and suddenly it's gone. I'm not accepting visitors, far less such hostile ones who haven't been invited. Clear off, I'm not ready yet.

Whilst jousting with the devil makes time pass more quickly, the rest of life is passing even faster. From keeping the finger on the pulse of my business to having absolutely no awareness of the wider world has been car-crash quick. There was plenty of work to do, people to contact and projects to complete without this interruption. Now there is the much bigger complication of handling enquiries from those to whom my absence is a real nuisance, as well as trying to succinctly explain what has happened to friends, long-lost buddies, relations and well-wishers.

Suzi is now everything to me: my ears, eyes, hands and mouth, as well as team cheerleader. In trying to make sense of all the surrounding chaos, she arranges visits by spreading out the numbers. Rather than allow the flurry of visitors from the first few days to continue, strict instructions are issued from our version of air traffic control. Like planes stacked to land at Heathrow, visitors will have to taxi, lest they clash with each other – or with one of the time-consuming nursing processes. Calls are transferred to her mobile phone and she garners email addresses to send out a regular Round Robin Update, pun intended.

Unfortunately, when sending out the first email Suzi announces she is now running my dairy. Requests for two pints of gold top go straight over our heads for the first few days until we realise the dyslexic howler. This doesn't augur well for explaining, let alone spelling or pronouncing Guillain-Barré correctly. By the way, it's Ghee-Yan Bah-Ray.

Then I receive a visit from the pain police. Yes, the hospital has an entire department dedicated to the study and relief of pain. Their leading professor, Michael, complete with silver beard and gravy-spattered tie, introduces himself as nonchalantly and sweetly as the arrival of apple blossom on a sun-kissed May morning. There is real kindness in this man, a reassuring tone to his measured words, and a Pandora-like ability to open my mind with a vocabulary previously unknown. Admittedly conversations are very one-sided, more monologue than verbal discourse, but his insights and past experience provide succour and balm.

Layer upon layer, he startes to build up a vivid picture of what it's like to be cast adrift inside this illness. His regular visits are supremely helpful. The body may be comatose but my mind is desperate for direction. He crafts words and sentences like a man working a block of wood, plying his rasp along the grain one moment then gouging feverishly the next. Michael has a remarkable ability to break complex emotions and behavioural study into memorable headlines. In such a woolly setting he provides clarity, reassurance and a sense of purpose. Not so much a strategy for recovery, more a hitchhiker's guide to redemption.

His visits starkly contrast with those of the gaggles of student doctors let loose across the ward. The unusual nature of my complaint means I'm a box office attraction. A senior physician assembles a posse of enthusiastic, dishevelled young people in white coats, talking to them openly about the patient in front of his or her bed as though that person doesn't exist. The hospital calls it the Committee Rounds. My reflexes have recently disappeared from my system and, as if to punish me for this crime, the student doctors are encouraged to lift my leg from the thigh upwards, strike me just below the knee with a specially adapted hammer as hard as possible and then watch in astonishment as absolutely nothing happens. They proceed to attack my ankle, elbow, wrist, and anywhere else they can think of, to witness the same compelling lack of movement.

As non-events go it's a good one, mirrored by my own muteness and inability to offer the merest hint of a bodily reaction. This stirs fresh animated discussion amongst the sartorially challenged committee, who confirm what a hopeless case I am. If the hierarchy of life resembles a food chain, their judgments, delivered in such a dismissive and insensitive way, demote me to the level of a not-so-fresh cabbage. Vegetables have feelings too, you know, and I want to cry like an onion. Yet I comfort myself with the knowledge that a committee is, after all, a group of the unwilling, picked from the unfit, to do the unnecessary. This makes me feel better, particularly because it's not fair or reasonable. But fair and reasonable are no longer part of my daily vocabulary. They've been replaced by words like nugatory and cadaverous.

CHAPTER SEVEN

Fall and Decline

Day 25 and the assault continues. Reports from the front line suggest new challenges are opening up. My hair is starting to fall out at an alarming rate, clumps of redundant silver decorating the pillow each morning. My bones are under threat of wasting like my muscles and need drugs to arrest this decline. Pain continues to escalate as my tolerance drops through the zero mark into negative territory. So I'm given a TENS machine to provide ameliorating electric impulses up and down my spine. Pregnant women will testify to the efficacy of the TENS system for suspending awareness of pain. It doesn't make it go away but it does at least screen some of the more malicious nerve tingles like a junk mail filter.

There's perverse news about my skin. My face is becoming blotchy and parched from lack of direct sunlight and due to my inability to process waste – it's blistering away as rapidly as if someone had set fire to it. But my body, until recently ripe with patches and scabs, is clearing up. The psoriasis is leaving its home because it needs a strong immune system to thrive and I'm no longer an attractive landlord.

My bottom meanwhile, in an act of genetic modification, has developed a satellite. Yes, I have grown a second sphincter. I feel surges of panic as each time I want to pass a stool, number one valve remains trenchantly closed while the new portal transmits 'mission accomplished' messages back to my disbelieving brain.

While all these problems, minor in themselves, are aggregating, I'm accumulating friendships with some of the nursing stars of the intensive care department who, it turns out, will remain constant in their companionship for months after I leave their care. I think it is more than pity. This 50th year, superficially so cruel in cutting me down to a very small size, is starting to offer an insight into the halcyon bits of human nature I always hoped would exist but which I've never witnessed. It's a veritable curate's egg of a year, indeed.

There are clear signs I have hitherto evaluated life with entirely the wrong gauge. This event has triggered such a tectonic split in the living experience that I'm now embarking on a second life on an entirely separate coastline. The sea of loss will always be there, cold, grey and as unforgiving as this storm's birthplace, yet the old order of things is gone for ever. The game of two halves is restarting with a fresh purpose.

Down in the murky depths of my decline, I land on a plateau. It lasts about a week. There is a lot to be said for plateaus. They offer familiarity, enabling you to become accustomed to your new-found circumstances. The fact that those circumstances are so absolute, so petrifying and so barren is not important. The lift is in the basement and can't descend any further. It brings new meaning to the idea of deep joy.

During this time the team experiment by increasing passages of time in which my breathing is less reliant on artificial support. They're trying to kick start my air consumption to make me independent again. Very short periods to begin with, measured in moments, lengthening each day.

My stomach returns to duty, reluctantly, and completes a half shift. It had become swollen and distended, constantly refilling with air, but now my pot-bellied pig profile slowly begins to defuse. The vocal cords are still mute, but I practise exaggerated enunciation, and those who spend most time with me learn, by lip reading, how to interpret more than one word in three.

Yet my limbs and muscles continue their route march to redundancy because there is no movement. So while part of my body considers an about-turn the rest remains in the exit marked stage left. This initial process of generating tiny improvements resembles archery practice. Concentrate on hitting the bull in the middle of the target – my body – and the cumulative score will rise with improvements in the stomach, spine and trunk.

To achieve full recovery, however, the analogy moves to the pub dartboard. You'll need to finish your game with doubles around the outside of the board – the fingertips and toes. These may remain isolated for years while the core of the body recovers. If you can't hit the double you'll be stuck until the day your whole being is reunited.

The point of intensive care is to stabilise patients as quickly as possible so they can be transferred into a specialist ward, making way for the next critical case. It's like Crewe railway station, an impressive structure that people frequently rush through, but definitely no corner table at Fortnum & Mason from which to gently while away the day.

I fervently believe that as I'm unable to do anything for myself I should remain in intensive care, hoping that – by divine intervention – I'll simply awaken one fine day, totally cured. The authorities know better though, and the boot camp regime begins in earnest.

The concept of physios trying to get movement out of a paralysed person may seem absurd, but that doesn't stop them coming each morning to coax me back into once familiar positions. It's vital work. There's so little that can be done with Guillain-Barré syndrome (GBS) sufferers by medicine or infusion that time and exercise are the only certain remedy. I try to join in as much as I can, but every piece of exercise creates untold pain. I'm plied with drugs to lessen the anguish but this merely reduces my squealing down to the level of a fractious banshee.

How disconcerting for the team to have their mitigating handiwork met with volleys of invective and tirades of rejecting noise. Articulate I'm not. So messed up are the signals from nerve end to brain that primal screaming is my only tongue. A new antediluvian language is being fabricated in the recesses of my vocal factory. Normal expressions like *Ouch* or *Urgh* are too ambitious, and cognitive thought a rarity, so finding appropriate grunts in lieu of language is as likely as striking gold on your first pan handle.

Better to imagine the world's worst audition for the job of backing vocalist to Manfred Mann's greatest hits – a veritable fusion of Doowaps, Doowadiddys,

Dididums and Didiyes sung by an urban fox on heat with the amplifier on distort. Or perhaps not. It's too depressing a thought – and thoughts and depression are becoming totally entwined.

Depression is an almost inevitable consequence of GBS so various concoctions are applied to find the optimum mix. This takes the edge off many things, particularly excessive fear, but eliminates the emotions at either end of the spectrum. It's a bit like removing both black and white to leave a palette comprising marginal changes in shades of grey. The upside is it stops you getting too depressed, the downside is that optimism is lessened, joy and euphoria removed. You trundle along in the middle lane of the carriageway.

Rational fear should dominate life. Fear of letting people down, of never realising the potential of a childhood rich in promise or of missing your own funeral. Fear of being permanently disabled or, even worse, of voting for the Liberal Democrats. Yet rational never answers the call. Opposite anxieties now take centre stage, trifling details about minutiae cramp my brain. All set against the certainty of my placement, flat on my back, six feet underground, denied energy, awareness and hitherto familiar reactions. The narcotics ensure my thoughts are surrounded and insulated by velleity, like an orbit in which a series of mild desires, wishes or urges are deemed too slight to lead to action.

And now the first 16 days of decline, post breathing collapse, have passed – just as the proverbial oil tanker is slowing before starting to turn – there comes a warning. We can't keep the bed available for you for much more than a month. After that you'll transfer into the neurology ward. The contrast between intensive care nursing, with one nurse per patient, to a department where one nurse looks after two bays of patients, will hit me hard. Apparently the experience will be like falling off the cliff at Beachy Head. I probably won't like it to begin with.

2

On the Ropes

A Solitary Confinement

- CHAPTER EIGHT -
On the Ropes

Sure enough, after 30 days, I'm transferred out of intensive care. I can now breathe unsupported for tiny moments – enough to justify my eviction. In short, I'm no longer sufficiently ill.

In their infinite wisdom the nurses decide to move me at 2am on a Sunday. I feel as though all the emotional crutches are being taken away at the same time, plus we can't stop off for a greasy kebab on the way, as men normally do at two in the morning after a Saturday night.

I'm placed into a neurological rehabilitation ward where they seem completely unfazed by my lack of animation. Patients with the movement of an Egyptian mummy waiting to be embalmed are evidently a way of life to the nurses and care workers who are to become my guardians and best friends for the next six months. Being paralysed, on a problem scale of 1 to 10, seems close to double digits to me. To the staff it's more a two or a three.

The new ward is full of old people. At least that's how it smells. I have no expectation of what a neurological ward will encompass. Principally it's where people who've had a first stroke go to recover. Or, and nobody ever talks about this, to wait for a second stroke which, if too soon after the first, can be really damaging, often fatal. I don't sleep that night. Or the next.

In fact it takes days to come to terms with my new surroundings. From my bed in the corner of the ward I should be able to keep an eye on all the other patients. Keeping an intermittent eye is all I can do. I can't sit up, let alone stand, and my powers of speech are still akin to the scoring of sandpaper on glass.

I'm actually in a prime position, with the most panoramic view of all goings-on. As my lumpy bed overlooks the other five bays, my job description is to be the new toll bridge teller, collecting fees from those who access or egress the ward. I can also see down two adjacent corridors and through an internal window over the L-shaped reception desk. It leaves very few hiding places for staff, patients or visitors. In this land of the blind the one-eyed man is king. King of Belvedere.

Strange how illness flattens us all and forges the most unlikely alliances. What's this? A youngster, or at least an arrival, that doesn't look like grandpa from a Werther's Original advert? The new bloke next to me used to stack the shelves at Sainsbury's during the night shift. He's 43 with two children, eight and five, and a particularly aggressive form of multiple sclerosis. A more giving person you could not hope to meet. Rapidly I become Butch Cassidy to his Sundance Kid. This is our tangent, where two seemingly unrelated people become one through adversity. How we will laugh at each other's misfortune, find solace in our ineptitude.

People keep coming and going from the bed opposite. Had they known its track record I'm sure none of those patients would have allowed themselves to be placed there. I watch 12 people die on that mattress right in front of me. They arrive off some magic conveyor belt which keeps churning out an inexhaustible supply of seriously ill patients with collapsed lungs, strokes down the left, strokes down the right, and organ failures. There are victims of badly administered drugs, negligent diagnoses, bad luck, and pneumonia or old age.

The first death is the worst. Nice enough fella… smoker, middle-aged and single – a stroke patient. Seems to be stabilising, then it all kicks off about one in the morning. Panic buttons, auxiliaries in scramble mode, zombie medics on their 14th hour of the day. The curtains fly open to shut, heart revival machinery is wheeled in. "Stay with us now, don't let go, hang on in there..." But it's to no avail.

I shall never forget the eerie sound of the first body bag being zipped up in the depth of the night, inch by uneven inch, while the night nurse sucks on her Murray mint. And yes, she takes her time. You never hurry a Murray.

It's a sound that makes you feel unclean.

In order to wash and change clothes it's necessary to be turned. Sometimes this is done by two or three staff working in a trained pattern. Remember

Cleopatra being delivered to the emperor by rolling out of the carpet across the marble floor? Now try to imagine her being wrapped into the carpet in the first place and you'll begin to understand what nursing teams do when caring for hopeless cases like me. They tug at my arms to create the momentum to flip me on to one side while lifting the base sheet across to the middle of the bed. They then roll me back on to my other side, removing the base sheet altogether.

Bed baths tend to involve two auxiliary nurses to wash you with tissues and towels, mild creams and occasionally stringent sprays. They work around the ward drawing curtains, before descending on the next patient. When wiping your bottom they're supposed to spray cleanser over you with the warning "cold spray!" Timing is never perfect however, and the spray tends to hit your nether regions long before the warning arrives.

It's not the best time for intimate reflection when one auxiliary nurse has just rolled you on to your tummy while the other tidies up your behind. I suppose we see a mild form of bottom interrogation when dogs sniff each other's backsides. We take this for granted while pretending to ignore the absurdity and obscenity of the pastiche, but this doesn't prepare you for the level of matter-of-fact attention your private parts receive in the course of a nurse's daily work.

Nor does it prepare you for the high speed with which you're returned to normal social etiquette. I wonder what the original *Sloane Ranger Handbook* would suggest as the most mannered way to show gratitude for having your arse wiped. I must ask the author next time I bump into him. Oh no, wait, there it is. Under Knightsbridge Girls: How to show gratitude. H is for help with ablutions, just after G for gang bangs… What's that? G is more interesting than H? Oh all right then. Aren't Knightsbridge Girls supposed to loathe gang bangs because they hate writing all those thank you letters?

Getting up and down to the toilet would, in a normal world, be an automatic process, but for the severely ill it's often impossible. So, under the influence of a mild anaesthetic, my plumbing has been readjusted. A bag is loosely strapped around my right leg just below the knee, and receives fluid through a pipe inserted into the eye of my penis. The bag is emptied periodically throughout the day. Some children have come to visit an immediate neighbour on the ward who is fitted with the same technology. With a splendid combination of spoonerism and malaprop, the youngsters invent a new term for the device. The *Catheteria*: a one-stop shop where you go for a pee and order a cappuccino at the same time.

Once inserted through the penis, a balloon attachment – at least ten times the size of the exit hole – is inflated inside the body to prevent the tube from being pulled out. I decide it's best to get on amicably with this new appliance and bedfellow. Others around me find this impossible. They wrench the device from their loins in an act of stupefying masochism. Either determined to ignore contrary advice, or unable to understand it, they scrabble away at themselves like kamikaze lemmings on a mission to remove the pipe. Oblivious to the pain they're about to cause, the yanking accelerates until their climactic howls of excruciation summon the nursing team to ease the agony and berate the patient for "being a pillock".

I resist the temptation to follow suit, partly because I've no desire to do it, partly because it seems absurdly painful and, of course, partly because I can't. Like most obstacles in life you overcome them and get used to them. Abdicating responsibility for another bodily function just means the list is getting longer. In time wearing a *catheteria* will matter to me and I'll want the faculty back, but at the present moment it's not even inconvenient.

Suzi provides so much cheer and practical help with basic ablutions that I don't know how anyone can manage without support from a loved one. By being at my side so unstintingly she replaces the nurses on countless occasions; or reminds them of tasks forgotten, or works with them as often two nurses are needed but only one available. They accept her as a member of the team, come to see her as part of their family and, dare I say it, come to take her help for granted while becoming very fond of her in the process. It's an act of unselfish dedication repeated daily and I'm humbled by her humanity, munificence and pluck.

The physio gathers pace incredibly slowly. I need to become used to life above the horizontal but the hare's approach is impossible when you can't even keep up with the tortoise. If you've ever tried moving a corpse you'll know how heavy a task it is to move a human being who can't co-operate. Getting anywhere near a sitting up position makes me dizzy, three pillows and I can't cope with the altitude. Sitting up on the edge of the bed is as intimidating as climbing the Eiger. I've no muscle control or strength, let alone the ability to stay unsupported in an upright position.

So I volunteer for more physio. You see, the NHS only offers physio from Monday to Friday. What I haven't appreciated before is that there are in fact two National Health Services: a weekday service and a weekend regime. On Mondays the wards overflow with doctors like a bountiful crop of strawberries spilling out of a punnet. As the week wears on their numbers dwindle. By Friday the exodus of expertise completes just before teatime. The result? Fridays are not a good day to be admitted to hospital – you're unlikely to receive any senior inspection until Monday. Indeed, Saturdays and Sundays feel like being aboard the *Marie Celeste*. It also seems that the worse your command of English the more likely you'll be on duty at weekends. Ill health doesn't recognise these barriers but they're there all right, entrenched like some unwritten apartheid.

I don't like the idea of a weekend devoid of effort to stimulate movement. It's a waste. To move away from my amorphous state I need to keep my body working seven days a week. The physios are, on the whole, very agreeable to extra weekend work in return for some pocket money. After a fight with my insurance company they agree to fund the cost and I start a grinding daily programme of minute improvement.

At best I can manage a half hour session because I've so little strength, but by gradually building up I'm eventually able to cope with more than one daily burst of activity. Day after day after day we go through the motions as I try to demonstrate enthusiasm and desire.

I have to learn the art of getting into and retaining a sitting position from scratch. My first attempt lasts precisely three seconds. One week of coercion later I'm ready for the next attempt. This lasts 30 whole seconds, providing the most fantastic endorphin-fuelled rush. Three days later I'm ready for the next bash and succeed in maintaining a position on the edge of the bed for two minutes unsupported. It's like winning the World Cup and drinking a bottle of vintage Krug all at the same time.

From such a lowly position the team drag me, always raising expectation and finding something positive to say, even when all the evidence is negative. I resemble an egg which needs its own carton to remain upright. Without it I find the line of least resistance, flopping or subsiding wherever gravity decides to take me.

I'm advised to talk to my limbs to send messages from the head to my extremities, nurturing the reflexes back to life. Well I send out the messages all right, in the vain hope some amateur radio ham will hear my mayday, tune in and broadcast a reaction back. This must be how a comedian feels when doing his first stand-up gig as a warm up for the main act. No one's listening, no one really cares, they just want the guy topping the bill to get on stage and make them laugh. It doesn't matter how good your script is, how much time you spend polishing and editing a razor sharp performance. If nobody wants to hear, then nobody will.

One of the things the doctor had told me about – which I hadn't really taken in after being poleaxed by the news that recovery would take two years – was my pain threshold, and how much worse things would get. In fact I've been reduced from having one to having less than none. Everything hurts.

Personally I prefer to have things suggested to me, not told in full. When every detail is given the mind rests satisfied and the imagination loses the desire to use its own wings. This is not good. My excruciating pain leaves no room for self-perfidy or for the mind to fly. It just continues to sharpen the poignancy, heighten the bittersweetness and drill right through my sense of enforced masochism.

Perhaps I'm becoming engulfed in thanatophobia, a morbid dread of death apparently universal in all except those living on Mount Olympus. I can't see Olympia or any Greek gods but I can see daffodils starting to appear outside the grubby windows. This makes me happier. Some days birdsong cuts across the acoustic medley of buzzers, bleepers and alarms, and some days we even see sunshine but still never a hint of those Greek gods.

CHAPTER NINE

On the Ropes

Pathos is everywhere, sad stories in front of your eyes of patients who don't know where they are, and worse still relatives who do not care. As spring arrives and the first tiny shoots of recovery in my body start to take hold, I feel like the elder statesman of the ward – if only because I've been there longer than anybody else and know how slippery the ropes can be for new recruits.

Each day I witness a vocabularical waltz between old Charles, on his fourth stroke, and his estranged wife who, like clockwork, appears at five to ten each morning armed with local newspapers. She's welcomed by vicious accusations of being late, wanton, slovenly and disloyal, and of forgetting his papers. She deflates this attack with calmness and serenity, reminding Charles she's five minutes early, has his newspapers and still loves him very much in spite of him being the most cantankerous old bugger she has ever met.

To say Charles is confused would do him a disservice. It's worse than that. His hearing is very poor, memory poorer still and, most terrible of all, he has lost the will to live – and to die. He sets off from his bed destined for the toilet but by the time he reaches the ward doorway can't remember why he set off in the first place.

One day the social worker comes to assess him. She pulls the soundproof curtains around his bed and begins asking questions. Charles can only conduct conversations at full volume so everybody else has no choice but to listen in.

"Do you know what year it is?" she enquires. "It ends in a three," he bellows. "Higher, higher," says the assembled audience of patients and nurses.

"Well, I'm not so sure, maybe it's four," Charles booms. "Higher, higher," urge the now enthralled game show devotees, giggling.

"Well, I think we've just had Christmas so maybe it's five," says Charles. Cue the most enormous cheer, wolf whistles, clapping, foot stamping and general revelry.

I've been able to witness this vignette while propped up. After what feels like months I'm beginning to sit up supported by two pillows. Now the physio team wants more. Its target is to get me into a wheelchair. Some days I doubt whether this will be achievable but it doesn't stop me trying. First I have to pass my hoist proficiency test so I can be lifted, like cargo from a ship's hold, high up into the air and rotated over the edge of the bed to be deposited on to trolleys, chairs or trestles before being winched back at a later time.

The bilious green hoist is tucked under my back and up through my legs. It's then clipped on to an electric pulley winched down from a track in the ceiling. Often this is the highlight of my day, particularly as it allows me to view the ward from a completely different angle. The joy of sitting upright fully supported, even if temporary, is a very real reminder of the liberty I've so completely surrendered.

Unfortunately it also offers a view of big John in the bed directly opposite. After suffering his second stroke, John somehow had managed to climb over the metal barriers attached on either side of his bed only to hit the floor with an almighty thwack, breaking his arm and dislocating his collarbone in one fell swoop. He's not an attractive man and has become prone to cussing and spitting. If his own plight has not already made him miserable, then the arrival of his family is sure to do it for him. In one of my least charitable moments I christen them the world's ugliest family, or the WUF for short. All of them – his eldest son, four daughters and one wife – have evidently finished the Atkins diet, and are now feverishly consuming *The Sumo Wrestler's Guide to Weight Gain*. Admittedly, physical criticism is a bit rich coming from me. I'm a 'Charles Atlas Before' advert with alligator skin, bald patches and feet shaped like inverted spoons, alongside fingers resembling the claw in the 'catch a cuddly toy' arcade machine at the end of Yarmouth pier.

But big John's family? A more unsavoury, malodorous and incipiently nasty group of people you could not hope to meet. They never engage in eye contact or conversation with any of the other relatives or patients. They constantly harangue and bicker with staff, are ungracious in the extreme and manage to get John's status relegated from one of sympathy to simmering contempt, crying wolf far too often on his behalf.

Resentful of the condescending way they're being treated, staff queue up to avoid looking after him, a soap opera that continues for several weeks. I grow tired of this little cameo and determine to intervene. Without uttering a word John and I develop a sign language using nods and winks, even the smile, so that I know when he's genuinely in trouble and really needs help. Some unwritten script entitles me to act as arbiter on his behalf. Bizarrely he receives attention if I indicate to the nurses with nudges and grimaces that this time his request is genuine.

Eventually he is transferred to another hospital, more akin to a hospice, and promptly replaced by a man whose troubles put everything else into perspective: Tom has motor neurone disease.

When first told that I had been diagnosed with GBS I was delighted because it wasn't the same illness as Tom's. My aunt had died from this slow, simmering, truculent affliction, and in my naivety I thought somehow it might have been genetically transferable. In the circumstances my lack of knowledge was inexcusable. Yet there I was, welcoming GBS like some lost friend, solely on the basis that it wasn't what I most feared.

Tom deserves better than that from me, he deserves better from life too. No one should have to suffer inside such an elongated death. He is a brave and noble man, stoical, fastidious and apparently completely lacking in self-pity. I salute him.

- CHAPTER TEN -

On the Ropes

O ften the best moments are surprises. One is on its way to meet me. I have no idea it's coming and don't think I'm anywhere near being ready. All that polished chrome, rich burgundy leather, go-faster wheels. Yes, it's time for the high back wheelchair.

All things are relative of course, so to someone unable to stir their carcass, a wheelchair is a tremendous statement of new-found mobility. To immediate family and helpers it offers something to do that demonstrates their support in a tangible way.

It's not easy to remain in. Yet the very fact my body is being put into and taken out of a wheelchair is therapeutic in itself. I can't say that I look forward to it – my spine is still too weak to support my body and my arms are unable to provide the ballast to stabilise me once in the chair. My head has to be tethered, my arms strapped over pillows at very specific angles, and my feet secured. It takes four people to get me in place, after getting me out of the hoist.

Somehow, each day, those four musketeers lever me into this unsuspecting wheelchair and strap me down to prevent my collapsing. It's torture, yet just a prelude to a more vertical challenge – learning to stand. I find the daily grind of trying to recover movement so tiring that I yawn during exercise. I have lost 3.5 stone and my body fat is down to Jane Fonda levels. Muscle, when idle, diminishes at about 3% per day. My arms are like twigs and I've been lying on my back far too long so my feet have dropped like a ballerina's. Now you may like a bit of foot action in *Swan Lake*, but I want to use them to stand.

Early lessons are to be conducted on a tilt table. I'm sure I saw something like this as a child on black and white television when an enigmatic man, dressed like William Tell, aimed his crossbow at the apple on the head of a glamorous assistant strapped to an upright tilt table with a look of foreboding on her face. I wear the same expression – but not the fishnet tights – and am petrified of tilting more than 45 degrees.

After multiple attempts which will eventually run to several months, we get the table up to 90 degrees. It feels as though I'm facing downwards, so strange is the sensation of being upright. My arms hurt in this position so I've a tray in front of me to keep my hands facing the horizontal. Every action seems to have a consequence involving pain. It never leaves. It's always there, gnawing at my resolve. But the conclusion is obvious. There is no substitute for simple hard work, if I'm ever to get better.

Meantime back in the ward, with a deft rotation of the beds, naughty Norman appears in the bay next to me. He's about 5' 3", blessed with long flowing white locks loosely arranged in the style of the first *Doctor Who*. If ever pyjamas were designed for one single human being it was Norman. A man born to wear jimjams, he has a cute pair of well-worn slippers and some well-worn stories too.

Poor Norman is losing his marbles. He needs help and far more understanding than is available on this ward. At night a film crew appears in his mind, provoking hours of in-depth interviews as he quizzes his alter ego. Innocent in the extreme, it's mildly amusing to begin with, but listening to the sadness of someone using an imaginary mobile phone with one voice to interrogate an illusionary person with a different accent and pitch became more and more harrowing. He has no recollection of what he has said over the last few moments or hours, nor any awareness of what constitutes night-time. There's some recollection of his youth but a ceiling came down about 30 years ago to wipe clean the memories in between. This is his second year of decline through Alzheimer's and Norman is living proof of how it's possible to be utterly alone even when surrounded by people.

From my world on a mattress the days pass and the weeks merge. Visitors arrive, by the yard. Some recoil in horror, others bring warmth and joy, but still they keep coming. I feel like King Canute, unable to overcome the invasion into my misery, but I realise that talking, or at least mouthing words, forces me to engage with the world, think of wider horizons and laugh at myself. So the visitors are essential to my recovery.

It was on an unsuspecting weekend that David B and Milena arrive with a humour so black my face aches with laughter. Pushing me out into the hospital's atrium coffee shop, my arms tied to the sides of the wheelchair, wrapped in swaddling blankets with my head leaning ominously to one side, I look like one of Jack Nicholson's finest *One Flew Over the Cuckoo's Nest* cameos. A pamphlet entitled *Sex After a Stroke* is placed under my chin, above a kidney bowl labelled 'Please Give Generously'. Off they tiptoe, leaving me alone as passing visitors try not to donate small change, while suppressing their grins.

I don't mind being laughed at but I do mind being surrounded by catering outlets. The exposure to food temptation is too much. I've not had a regular meal since admission, and my taste buds are grateful to have escaped the enticement of seasoning and flavour. I will need to relearn the skills and pleasure of consumption.

That night David B, from my bedside, tries to book a table for dinner in 27 restaurants, all of which are full, before finally finding one with an available table. As he confirms the timing the waiter is surprised to learn he wants a table for three, for this is Valentine's night (a date David has completely overlooked). As he puts down the handset, David hears the waiter softly breathe one condemning word, "pervert". Which, of course, makes the dinner delicious for me.

My previous world of lunch and supper is about to mutate into a new northern land where dinner is at midday, tea at five and Maltesers with my fellow inmates, such as Butch and Sundance, munched at any time. Chocolates and sweets are becoming our currency, preferably in a stolen moment when no one is looking or counting our blood sugar level.

Amidst all these nasty manifestations of illness – strokes, heart arrests and the like – there is a quiet and ruthless predator at work. Diabetes is an odious, pernicious invader of our systems borne out of our 21st century lifestyles. Ignorance is its ally, constantly aiding and abetting. Top tip: don't fill your blood with sugar.

I choose to ignore all this incredibly sensible advice as I lie quiescent on my bed mouthing "yes please" when Sundance asks if I'd like another Malteser. I can move my mouth about two inches to either side and one inch up and down, which doesn't help my chances of catching anything. For Sundance, whose legs are wobbly and whose arms don't work too well, keeping the Malteser bag in an upright position takes a lot of concentration. It's quite likely he'll fall over in the process.

Sundance, however, is determined to get one of the brown sweets into my mouth. It's necessary for him to drop them from a great height to maintain his balance, which doesn't help target practice or the laundry bill. At the 12th attempt we manage a hole in one, but at some cost. Chocolate blobs are everywhere, in the sheets, on the floor and inside my pyjamas – there are even two in the bedpan.

Trying to eat cake is almost as difficult as trying to hide the evidence of my snacking. No matter how strong my denial, the residue of crumbs in the armpits always gives me away. Out of sight is out of mind, though, and as I can't adjust my head to look down the bed to witness the flaky evidence, I can carry on defying diabetes to my heart's content.

One of the consequences of remaining supine is that haircuts become hazardous. The hospital employs a roving hairdresser who weaves between the wards, offering trims and rinses to as many customers as she can fit into one day. My hair hasn't been washed for two months or cut for three; the words *bouquet like an Aborigine's armpit* do little justice to the steamy halo that welcomes this intrepid crimper.

Unable to get me into a sitting position she cuts my hair horizontally. The result is memorable, particularly for those unfortunate enough to have to look at me. Boris Karloff would have been proud. As I can't look into a mirror I'm not too bothered. Initially. Indeed, if I don't want to talk to somebody it's a positive advantage as patients and visitors veer off in opposite directions trying to mask their contempt.

This merriment of the mullet continues until an old Sicilian is admitted to one of the ward beds. Joe senior, who moved to this country more than a generation ago, has just experienced a second stroke, leaving him unable to speak and more flatulant than any man I've ever met. Admittedly I used to play rugby in the second row with a bloke whose post-match party piece was to fart at will. He could cluster them, broadcast them in stereo and, after a few pints of Bass, stop all conversation by firing off a salvo from the heart of his bottom (guaranteed to clear the bar). Nobody ever needed to ask why he was called Gatling.

But Joe's family used to visit him in the classic Italian way. First the mommas and the poppas, then the sons and daughters, closely followed by the grandchildren and their babies. No one else commands such an audience by saying so little, to such a wide variety of relations. The rest of the patients pray for them to stay for as long as possible as their endless Sicilian/English chatter sounds so peaceful in comparison with the crescendo we all know will surely follow after the family's mass departure.

As the last "ciao!" subsides Joe starts to crank up the volume from underneath the sheets. This is Premier League farting, no nationwide conference part-time bottom burping here. Wilfred Owen would have been proud of the onomatopoeia, as one 'Rat a ta tat' rolls into the next 'Rat a ta tat'. I swear I can hear a descant in there somewhere. On one particular occasion the man in the bed next to me starts singing a song once famous as the accompaniment to a *Real Thing Coca-Cola* advert: "I'd like to teach my bum to sing, in perfect harmony." Although I confess, it's just possible these may not have been the exact lyrics – and the singer might be me.

Joe's son, Joe Junior, unaware of the flatulent opera that takes place each night after he leaves, is overheard opining on the state of my haircut from across the ward. After 25 years in this country he speaks a curious mix of English which most closely resembles Stavros, Harry Enfield's Turkish kebab shop owner. There's a burr of West Country, plenty of Italian and even a bit of north London cockney as Joe utters the memorable lines: "Jesus Christ, look at the state of that bloke's barnet, it's in a right two and eight and no mistake."

He comes over to talk to me. "Listen mate, no offence but your 'ead is making me sad. I'm a 'airdresser, and I fix it for you." Next day he arrives with his mother and proceeds to give me a tip top haircut. After we've exhausted the usual banter about "Where you going on your 'olidays?" Joe starts to wax lyrical about his four daughters. It's as though he's announcing the winner of the Miss World competition as he explains to me how wonderful each one is in reverse order.

There's nothing too surprising about the choice of language to describe the majesty of each of his girls, but as he snips away he's clearly building up to a crescendo. At last we get to the beauty of the eldest, who, like the other three, works with him in the salon. I'm expecting a word like *bellissimo* as Joe details her long dark hair, curvaceous hips, winning smile and knowing look. "My first daughter, she is, how you say? A right belter."

He's not wrong. She's stunning and it's absolutely the last time I expect to hear a father describe his daughter so cutely or curiously. His mother ignores us and carries on sweeping up the hair cuttings from the floor.

Life is not just focused on the hair on my head though. There are other hairy bits to consider. "How is your erectile function?" enquires the immaculately groomed doctor who has recently given birth to an immacutely groomed baby daughter. Attractive, with a confidence, quick brain, trim figure and air of immense capability, she's not the sort of woman you can imagine cracking nudge nudge jokes with. This doesn't stop me trying a self-mocking riposte. Fortunately it gets strangled somewhere in my vocal chords. It's not a question I've considered or encountered before.

Do you consider this to be a closed question, implying a single word response? As in "fine" or "disastrous". Even more damning, I suppose, could be the multiple choice option, "don't know". It's possible to go for the more expansive explanation, assume it's an open question and that the doctor has a spare half hour for you to pontificate ad nauseam on the vacillations of your willy. In the end I opt for the medium response, mumbling, "I think there's still a bit of life there." Which may well be true. The trouble is that at this particular moment I can't remember and my body has stopped sending me updates.

Try it at dinner parties. Not at the start of the evening, I grant you, but after dessert when the cognac is being proffered. It's a killer question and I promise none of your guests will ever forget the evening, or forget to consult that *Sloane Ranger Handbook* to check how best to construct their thank you letters. Have a look, it's probably in there under E.

3

Shoots of Recovery

A Solitary Confinement

CHAPTER ELEVEN

Shoots of Recovery

After the daffodils comes Easter. The view out of the ward windows, on the few days when warm clear sunshine bursts through, are now of scaffolding against tired redundant buildings. Normally clad by sublimely coloured stone in shades of cinnamon, the empty properties are reduced to tawdry ochres, anthracite greys and dust-covered piles of rubble. The trust in charge of the hospital's finances are splashing out on bigger corridors for all, while awaiting the arrival of their fourth chief executive in three years.

The rose garden beckons. An area of peace and calm sheltered from the wind, it's a sanctuary in which to revive the soul. How I look forward to those moments when I can feel the sun on my face, and the spirits rise. The sunshine brings both relief and expectancy. The realisation starts to surface that, after four months, I might indeed be able to get better, while my determination to conquer the illness strengthens when outdoors.

The garden is in a courtyard, two sides created by the walls of the original 1930s hospital, the other two by glazed corridors leading to the children's ward. It's difficult for the wind to circulate too close to the ground – and certainly at wheelchair height – but no matter how seductive the sunny days appear, it's the time of year when bitter cold can cut to the bone, turning a potentially pleasant afternoon sojourn into *Ice Station Zebra*. A central fountain which provides an ideal bird bath for ravens and seagulls is surrounded by four oblongs of earth planted with roses of all primary colours. In true municipal planting fashion the colours clash horribly. Who invented the rule that any exposure to civic planting should attack one's eyesight so spitefully?

Garden maintenance is not high on the hospital's budgetary concerns, so for much of the year it lies untended, save for the magpies raiding the waste paper bins and leaving a trail of debris. Miraculously the garden's borders sport herbaceous arrays in which some emotionally intelligent soul, blessed with an awareness of how to blend colours and tones, has laid out shrubs and flowers with delicacy and great care. There's the usual mixed bag of benches donated by grateful relatives, dedicated to departed loved ones. Above and behind these are bushes, plants and trees including the most delightful *Paulownia tomentosa*, a tree of Chinese extraction boasting a trumpet-shaped lilac flower, with branches weeping down over the east corner.

There's a certain air of *The Secret Garden* attached to this space. So few people know of its existence, or, if they do, they're blind to its charms. I'm not very keen to share the secret, a selfish emotion I know, but one of its many-faceted attractions is the solitude and silence. A sylvan sense of nature embraces you. Reminders of the countryside's charm pervade and help provide equilibrium to my mind, something my troubled carcass is unable to do.

Without such respite the ward's immediate surrounds force melancholia on all of us. They confront us with the one truly philosophical problem. You know… suicide, judging whether life is or is not worth living. To answer this is to answer the fundamental question of philosophy – and I can tell you without equivocation the answer is 'yes'. For I'm far from alone, and surrounded by too many strident examples of optimism, to dwell too long in such torpid isolation to toy with the 'no' word. Besides, Suzi will never give me permission.

Amidst the sadness of ill health there are people who work every day helping the nurses to get people better. Auxiliary Care Helpers, with their deprecatory humour and readiness to do difficult, awkward and menial tasks, make me realise just how lucky I am to have spent so much time working under the comfort blanket of palatial hotels. My career had suitably servile beginnings, but I rose through the ranks to become an owner and operator of hotels with the sort of character, facilities and style customers dream of staying in. This allowed me to live like a millionaire, bypassing the need to become one. Need a Diet Coke at 2am? Just dial room service.

What bitter irony that I should have devoted so much time catering for generally self-obsessed people to whom staying in posh hotels became a right, putting their happiness ahead of mine. Because now the role is wholly reversed and I, the selfish customer, don't just need Coke at 2am, I need to receive dedication from anyone who'll pay attention.

How I rejoice when, one fine morning, Rupert from bed 6 strides across the ward to the reception desk dragging his catheter trolley behind him and announces: "I wish to check out. Please prepare the bill and have the car brought to the front." They tranquillise him and put him back to bed. He dies the next day. The bill remains unpaid in one way, but at far too high a price in another.

The nurses, it increasingly appears, dish out the drugs while the care workers wash me, carry me, dress me, feed me, nurture me and never make me feel as though I'm asking too much. For their collective strength and individual humility I shall always be grateful. Of course there are stars but all are special people. Very special.

There's an expression which now pervades the NHS and supposedly sums up a perceived malaise. Apparently present-day nurses are 'too posh to wash', leaving the lion's share of the duties to the care workers, in theory the least trained and qualified staff. This may be true, but what I perceive is that whenever the teams work together as one unit, with purpose, the patients get looked after more quickly, the general mood is lighter and there always seems to be time to spare. When those members of the brigade more obsessed with hierarchy take charge, anarchy breaks out in the ranks, less work gets done, patients are more at risk and a sense of unrest hangs uneasily in the air.

Behind most major illnesses today are a number of charities, trusts and supporting bodies. It's still a surprise, however, to find that such a little-known ailment as mine possesses such wide-ranging help. The GBS Association has set up a voluntary support group and once added a green tortoise to its logo. It's almost entirely composed of volunteers with past experience of the illness.

I'm fortunate to come under the guiding wing of John Beaven. A local journalist who had fallen prey to the syndrome some five years ago, John has made a full recovery save some tingling in his feet. Armed with the most considerate manner he visits me once a week, never overstaying his welcome and always prepared with advice appropriate to the next stage of my recovery.

His pastoral care is an elixir. It's a privilege to know him and a permanent bond is burned deep inside. That he should call from his annual holiday in France to check on my welfare speaks volumes for the quality of the man.

To our delight and surprise we realise our parallel lives have crossed before. Some 20 years previously I'd sat next to his wife at dinner in the Cotswolds. We shared a passion for Bath Rugby Club's many triumphs (and escalating list of inglorious moments) and one of my oldest pals worked with him at the same local newspaper desk for five years. He'd covered all the winter sports, and one other in particular that takes place from April to September. Yes, with spring comes cricket.

The local ground is adjacent to the hospital. Known as the Lansdown Cricket Club, it's where the great Sir Vivian Richards made his debut in England. It's also where helicopters land with Accident and Emergency cases from surrounding counties. Although the pitch doesn't have quite the same history or romance as Canterbury, Kent's county ground, where an antique oak tree stands within the white boundary rope – if your stroke hits it on the full you score a unique six – it certainly has its protocol. No matter how delicately poised the match, play is interrupted the moment players or umpire hear the whir of helicopter rotor blades. If the bowler has started his run-up, the delivery is completed – and the rest of the over suspended – while the players retire to the clubhouse.

As the indigo blue ambulance helicopter draws near, scattering spectators in its wake, the emergency team rushes out with its stretcher trolleys and draws as close to the circumference of the rotating blades as it dares. It's quite a spectacle. Critical cases from all over Gloucestershire, Somerset, Wiltshire, Devon and Dorset are regularly rushed expeditiously into the womb of the intensive care unit.

Once the helicopter sets off on its next mission and a prudent interval has passed, play resumes as tenaciously as before. The quality of games varies enormously. Sometimes an ex-England fast bowler opens the attack, at other times a novice 11-year-old, without hand-to-eye co-ordination, closes it all too quickly. Why, even the ladies get in on the act.

Strapped into my wheelchair, Suzi and I potter along the corridors away from the ward to while away 30 minutes watching matches. As my confidence grows,

I graduate to a crafty half-pint of beer from the white timbered clubhouse. The first taste is like a magical elixir, once familiar hops, barley, malt and subtle fragrances shock the palate, for so long rendered redundant, now electrocuted back to sparkling life.

My arms still don't work, but the pain is shifting from my body, millimetre by millimetre. The spine, which had been in the most intense agony, has recovered some feeling and strength. Yes, my arms and legs remain unimpressed at the prospect of any work and my hands never stop hurting in the most aggressive fashion, but once you become used to the pain you accept it as part of your daily life.

The sense of helplessness is still all-engulfing. Apart from being able to move my head from side to side and open and close my mouth and eyes, there's little other movement I can initiate, or congruous sound I can project. There are still too few reasons why anyone should want to talk to me. However, my one-way conversations – the most restorative medicine so far – are increasingly becoming close to two-way. I 'chat' with nurses, fielders at silly mid on, care workers, Suzi (always) and my family of philanthropic friends. It's progress. Clear progress.

- CHAPTER TWELVE -
Shoots of Recovery

Springtime is proving to be an inspiration. It brings variety, a change of scene, and it encourages movement. Perfecting my standing to begin walking becomes the next objective. Now I've learned to be upright on a tilt table, the next frontier is the hydrotherapy pool. It helps my flexibility and enables me to stand and take the faintest steps supported by water.

It seemes so liberating – until, that is, I meet Kirsten's breasts. With great generosity, it seems to me, she fills her swimming costume in the most ample way. Proportions become vital, although relative. At 5' 1" she's 14 inches shorter than I am, so there's no justifiable reason why my chin should be so inexorably attracted, apparently by magnetic force, to her bosom. But there my chin hovers, dipping and diving in one convulsion after the next as I struggle manfully to unfurl my spine and stand to attention (in the non-biblical sense). I will always maintain I owe my ability to straighten up to these watery encounters.

Getting in and out of the pool is quite a performance. A crane carries a specially adapted chair up and over the water in an arc before lowering the incumbent into the over-chlorinated depths. Thirty six degrees centigrade is a lovely temperature and essential for people like me with poor circulation. For 20 blissful minutes I lurch around supported by two members of the physio team who understand how likely it is that I'll capsize. I don't let them down. Those early moments enable me to practise my arctic roll over and over again, so I'm ready to start advanced canoeing lessons the very next day.

Shamelessly I'm savouring these moments as the centre of attention. The illusion is shattered when the first member of *The Cripples' Fat Club*, as they introduce themselves, enter the water with me. She's followed by 12 more people over the next five minutes who invade the water in a variety of ungainly ways. Each has suffered some debilitating problem either from an accident or neurological attack. They look as elegant as a daddy long legs after some recalcitrant child has sadistically pulled off several limbs. All are grotesquely overweight and, once in the water, bob up and down, minimising their efforts to burn off calories and improve mobility. They just wanted to talk – it's like an aquatic coffee morning. The only part of their physique to receive any material exercise is the jawbone.

It's impossible not to get in their way but I'm not interested in giving up my moments in the pool. The sensation of warm water on the flesh and the opportunity to defy conventional gravity are so rewarding. I'm reminding my muscles of the sort of work that they used to do, a refresher course of paramount importance. I'd happily have spent all day, every day in that pool in spite of the fellow attendees. Sadly I can only visit twice a week, the control of visiting times is democratic, and many patients have equal need.

Meanwhile, the status quo in my throat has begun to change. I've been unable to project my voice for more weeks than I care to remember, resorting to exaggerated movements of the lips and inviting any listener to get as close to my face as they can bear. It's extraordinarily frustrating for both parties. Inevitably you end up repeating statements and requests several times, without understanding what it is in your delivery that the person cannot grasp. Some nurses seem to have a special antenna, enabling them to tune in immediately, barely missing a word. Others might as well be studying Esperanto.

Curiously, the most attentive are the Spanish nursing staff. Out of roughly 1,200 full-time hospital employees, 108 are from Spain. Evidently their medical training system creates too many applicants for too few jobs. So their health authorities have gone into the export market and the United Kingdom is happy to oblige. The Spaniards arrive with finely honed nursing skills and a mixed bag of 'wordsmithing' abilities.

The one first assigned to me is called Manuel, all the way from Barcelona. A tall, handsome and charming 21-year-old, he only needs to look at a girl for her to understand any language he chooses. He and his compatriots are so used to asking people to repeat themselves to help improve their language, understanding me does not seem so difficult. After all, I already have to enunciate slowly and with great exaggeration. I must remind them of their early language tapes when they tried to comprehend our fascination with 'The Rain In Spain Staying Mainly On The Plain'.

The sinister rasping which escapes my throat whenever I try to speak comes from my need to exhale words rather than inhale them. It's extraordinarily stressful and tiring because the neck muscles are so reduced and my lung power minimal. Humans speak with remarkable laxness and imprecision, yet we express ourselves with subtlety at breathtaking speed – around 300 syllables a minute in normal speech. After forcing air up through the larynx we then purse our lips and flap our tongue to shape the passing puff of air into loosely differentiated plosives, fricatives and gutturals, which emerge as a more or less continuous wall of sound. We Do Not Talk Like This, wetalklikethis.

Are you following? It helps to picture a watercolour painting left out in the rain. Just as the colours run together, so do our syllables, words and sentences. Getting the words on to the painting in the first place means practice and patience, for voluble I'm not, nor pleonastic. Mellifluous, that's how I want to be, no matter how many duff paintings I create on the way.

For those stroke victims around me, struck down the right side of their bodies, speech is a real difficulty. Learning how to use your second hand late on in life is difficult enough, but expressing yourself with severely or permanently compromised speech is something I can't comprehend, far less accept.

My body, though, is learning new alternative ways to express itself, particularly through my recovering appetite. Is it magic, centrifugal force, or willpower that keeps me upright in the swimming pool? It certainly isn't a balanced nutritional diet. The hospital offers a three-week rotating menu which remains unchanged whatever the season. There are all kinds of pies: fish pies, ocean pies, shepherd's pies, pies from cottages, and *Spécialité de la Maison* exhausted steak without any kidney pies. Even without the muscle-wasting illness, the lack of intellect in the planning of the NHS menus means my chances of recovery are severely compromised.

Continuing to serve food from a hospital cook-chill menu so mundane, so lacking in aspiration, so contemptible should be a hanging offence. I've lost weight at a spectacular pace, dropping from 15 stone to 11½ stone. I hold out no prospect of gain with this pie-in-the-sky diet.

CHAPTER THIRTEEN

Shoots of Recovery

Amidst all this ribald entertainment, occupying the mind becomes more important. So I attempt to graduate from counting the panels in the ceiling, through trying to remember the names of all the staff, to listening to audiotapes. Ricky Tomlinson is my favourite. He tells his life history from casual entertainer, through picket on lightning strike and a spell in prison, to his finest hour: encouraging the nation to say 'My Arse' while sitting in a big armchair in the classic sitcom, *The Royle Family*. There's something sad yet encouraging about his Liverpool tones, and something so wonderfully Scouse about his excuse that everything is always someone else's fault.

So what about me? I've been trying to work out who's at fault in my own case. Admittedly, the previous year had been quite stressful, a deal had taken too long to complete, and certain projects been slow to progress. But what have I done wrong? Who's to blame? Could I have done things differently?

Question after endless question revolve around the bedside, but I can't come up with an answer. The purchase of London's premier club-cum-hotel, Home House, had been completed on 6th December, two weeks prior to my falling ill. It was a long and protracted process, spread out over an entire year, placing a considerable strain on our team. The lawyers had a field day and we hit many points when giving up seemed the only sane option. I'm delighted we didn't – the business is quite unique and has grown strongly since – but the stress of chasing the deal was nothing so out of the ordinary that it should single-handedly cause a collapse like mine. I had just turned 50 and hoped this would be a year of milk and honey. Then it vanished.

But I'm the lucky one. I have a return ticket. Every other patient I meet has a new level of compromise in their life and has only booked a single flight. Motor neurone disease, cerebral palsy, ME and MS, meningitis, stroke, aneurysm, these are the stock ingredients. Or how about septicaemia, major organ failure plus heart surgery, sprinkled with nutmeg and topped with a final burst of Guillain-Barré, for good measure? Oh, I nearly forgot, Mike Harvey – a brother-in-arms from college days – was in a coma for months as well. But more of him later.

Whenever I start to feel sorry for myself I have to stop. It isn't realistic to harbour petty jealousies when I'm surrounded by people so much worse off than me. My lifeline has always been, and remains, hope. Hope that things will improve. Hope that there will be a next stage to life worth looking forward to. Hope that there might be a regime beyond faith and charity. Yet faith and charity provide the only embrace to so many of my companions. "He that is down needs fear no fall, he that is low needs fear no pride," says Gabriel, my neighbour in bed 4. They are the last words he speaks to me, or anyone for that matter, as he never wakes up again.

In some cases the state of the visitors appears even worse than that of the patients. One particular father had been battling cancer for many years only to be struck down with a heart attack leaving his mouth skewed at a funny angle and removing most of his speech faculty. His dutiful wife visits every day and is so used to the hospital environment that she's completely unfazed by the surroundings.

Their sons, though, are a mixed bag. The eldest had a car accident which broke many of his bones before the car burst into flames, setting fire to most of his body. It's quite miraculous he's alive and even more staggering that his spirit remains so content. He matches this with a genuine concern for others and refusal to be broken. Looking in the mirror each day must be a constant reminder of the agony and devastation the accident has wrought.

The middle son, meanwhile, has a scary form of gigantism, enlarging his bones in awkward places. His hand span is quite disproportionate to the rest of his frame, his eyes pop out of his head as if attached on stalks.

The youngest has inherited the good looks, eye for the ball and silver tongue along with all the good genes going. With such a head start you'd expect him to be the Samson of the family, taking the collective weight on his shoulders. Unfortunately there's an addictive side to his personality and he invariably turns up to visit his father drunk as a lord.

None of this stops dad sharing out his love equally among his boys. Although bound by the vows of silence his illness imposes, he still communicates his affection by gesture, lopsided smile and hearty laugh. This man has been in and out of hospital for years, and his wife can barely remember the last time they enjoyed life without such enduring obstacles.

How I wish for special magical powers to provide them with the alchemy to reprogramme and vivify their flawed destiny. After all, I've previously developed a soft drinks business making specials for high street notables with flavours ranging from elderflower, lime, grape and apple to lemon grass, schisandra, ginko and echinacea, so blending things comes easily to me. Or at least it used to. That was the old, genial, gregarious me. Now I'm an island – a Robinson Crusoe on Friday's day off – living in mental isolation in vituperative ignorance, unaware of my effect. So I've no idea of the tragic figure I present to them. For all my sympathy, they return the affection with interest. While I cry for them, in their eyes my story is every bit as woeful.

I close mine to hide the tears, hoping to drift off to sleep before the late shift clocks on. I don't succeed. The ward teams work in three eight-hour shifts, rotating through early, late and night. Most staff work a combination of all three, a few only work days but the SAS storm troopers just do the nightshift. These are the hardy souls, who balance gloom and doom with a raucous sense of mischief. I give them nicknames, of which they know nothing.

Blofeld is the first, a cheerful lad who lives on a farm by day, treats me like someone he can talk to but is wrapped up in his plans to get married on the seventh of the seventh month in 007. Can I help him find an Aston Martin to be the wedding car? Of course, I want to say. Pass me my jacket, there's one in my coat pocket.

Yogi is, inevitably, a bear of a man, as wide as he is tall, with the strength of a shire horse and surprisingly cerebral personality. He overhears *If* by Rudyard

Kipling – I've now turned to poetry for my easy listening – and immediately turns the volume down to recite the words directly to me. Where it takes three nurses to adjust my position, it needs just one tug of his strong arm to yank me back up the bed. His surfeit of strength gives me vicarious pleasure. What energy I have left seems just out of reach. It has exited at such speed, and hasn't left a forwarding address.

The Jailer is an altogether different specimen. How she has become a nurse I'll never know. She has the perfect personality to work on the complaints desk at Easy Jet. Loud, vulgar, abusive and hungry, she skips her duties as quickly as possible so she can open a can of Coke and wade her way through the first of her Indian or Chinese takeaways, belching with sapient delight. Each night you pray someone else will be allocated to look after you. Somewhere inside this termagant must be a caring soul but my goodness, how hard she fights to hide it. The jangle of the Jailer's keys will stay with me for a long time. I may never forget it.

Meanwhile, back on the day shift, the person opposite me wants a fag. His lungs have collapsed, he's coughing up blood and he's just had a heart attack – a mere inconvenience delaying the next cigarette. Many patients head outside the hospital in their fluffy slippers, pushing intravenous drips on chrome trollies, to join their relatives puffing away at little white sticks as if winning the lottery depends on the next drag. In sub-zero temperatures women, plumbed into their catheter bags and wrapped in hospital nightgowns, gather in a tribal ritual outside the smokers' shelter. It doesn't matter how much rain or snow is falling. They stay outside because inside stinks of stale cigarettes. Not one of them finds this ironic, nor, more importantly, cares what they're doing to their health; the tobacco addiction is in absolute control.

Maybe, just maybe, there is a link between our health and our behaviour. I've already decided there must be, so seek out any assistance to get me better. In addition to helping me relearn the art of standing in the pool, a galaxy of implements and devices are incorporated into my daily routine. At night my feet are placed into plaster casts to reduce the effect of the foot drop. The casts, made on-site to order, are rebuilt every three weeks to encourage the rake of my feet to return to a position close to a 90-degree angle to my shin. By day splints are placed around my ankles and hamstrings to help me stand and lift my feet.

Indeed, every physio session aims to make me comfortable with sitting up, then standing, then walking. To get from a sitting position on the edge of the bed into a wheelchair the team take me to the gym and upgrade me to a banana board: a piece of wood shaped into a curved L. Half of this is shoved underneath one buttock on the side of the bed, leaving the other half projecting over the wheelchair. One of the chair's armrests is removed allowing you to slide across the board and into the seat. It requires considerable focus from the physios and a series of bunny hops from the patient. It sounds so simple but to me is incredibly difficult. Preparing for each hop, which at best moves me a couple of inches, requires similar focus and effort to running down the track in the Olympic pole vault.

My arms still appear to have nothing to give and my fingers hurt like hell. The occupational therapy team, led by the lithe and deceptively strong Shona, massage my hands every day. You need a microscope to see any improvement but that doesn't stop us looking. The manipulation of my hands provides temporary relief and miraculously uncovers the tiniest movements. The little finger on my left hand can wiggle from side to side. Hallelujah! It can't go up or down or turn but it's a start. The middle finger of my right hand starts to straighten but the muscle has eroded completely, leaving loose flesh in all its wasted glory hanging between each digit. Without prompting, these skeleton hands curl inwards forming a curious and sinister claw. Hand splints are supplied to be worn at night – and whenever resting by day – to help the wrist, palm and fingers rediscover a more normal position. There's nothing spectacular about these incremental steps which proffer no more than marginal improvement. It's a slog.

Fortunately the hospital possesses a hi-tech kit promising cumulative benefit from a very meagre beginning. By embracing it from the third week of May, I accelerate my recovery along with the volume of muscle repetitions I can achieve in any one day without my legs completely giving up. The wondrous battery-powered portable contraption 'super-assists' my attempts to complete mission impossible: standing up.

Specious in a shocking livery of purple, yellow and grey, the Arjo Encore – a sort of minitaure forklift truck – becomes my 'must have' travel companion. I sit on the edge of the bed as the Arjo is wheeled backwards towards me. My feet are placed on to its plinths and a belt wrapped around my middle and held in place by a rigging system clearly designed by a yacht builder. In fact, using it brings back memories of my first attempts at waterskiing. My hands are strapped on to two metal levers which rise upwards as the belt pulls me inexorably towards the main shaft of the machine, leaving me with no option but to achieve a standing to attention pose.

Well that's the theory. The practice proves very different. The levers haul my arms up all right, the belt digs into my buttocks to shift my frame, and the machinery drags the legs up into the air. So far so good, except for my right ankle which turns outwards, taking all of my weight through it once I'm fully upright. Without the reflexes to shift my weight to my left side I can only react by exhaling belly grunts of displeasure. These are not cries of pain, they're worse than that. Far worse. I sound like a sea lion berating a mate. You might think I'm making a fuss but it leaves me unable to stand properly on my right leg for three weeks – even with the balm of cold compresses, regular physiotherapy and acupuncture.

If it's this difficult for me, goodness knows how someone like Douglas Bader was able to cope. If he could learn to walk again without his own legs and start to play golf to a decent standard then I'm not going to let this be anything other than a minor setback. The good news is that my muscle memory loss is so close to absolute that one day I might relearn golf without retaining all those unreliable habits I've added to my haphazard game over too many years.

With that in mind, this appears to be the perfect moment to try some fairway striding exercises. Cometh the hour cometh the harness. The system was dreamt up by the head physio who, without realising it, has become my hero. Kirsten has the gift of being able to make you do things your body doesn't want to do, more often than you ever believed possible, and to repeat the exercise the next day. Somehow she makes it pleasurable.

Like a young child's first pair of dungarees, the harness – attached to a track in the ceiling of a vacant ward – is wrapped around my chest and groin as I sit in the wheelchair. Slowly it, and therefore I, am winched upwards from my wheelchair until my legs are straight. I can now raise my left one an inch or so, just enough to begin the process of walking. The right leg does not want to join in however, and trails behind like Quasimodo's haunches. In front of me I have a tall frame on wheels, which allows me to rest my arms, dubbed the pulpit. Within seconds I'm too out of breath to deliver a sermon but, with a great deal of coaxing, manage ten paces before collapsing quite exhausted. The following day we manage 12 paces. And so the process continues.

"Kick out like an ostrich!" comes the instruction. Apparently ostriches splay their feet when they walk. This makes me want to sing. So there we are, two physio instructors and I, lurching across the floor with my left foot splayed, Quasimodo's right dragging behind, singing *Springtime for Hitler and Germany*. Yes, *The Producers* have arrived all the way from Broadway. Admittedly we don't manage the goose step on day one but most mornings bring some marginal improvement and, after a month or so, I'm ready for the pulpit without the harness. My groin's in ecstasy at this development. Weeks of the 'dungaree nether regions' have forced me to sing springtime in falsetto. Now I can tackle baritone.

By putting pressure down through the elbows I'm able to take some weight on to the pulpit, giving my legs a chance of bearing the rest of me. I've some limited strength in my shoulders and the top of my triceps, none in my biceps or any part of my hand or forearm, but it's a start. Goodness knows how toddlers manage. I don't remember it seeming such hard work at their age. An hour of this a day is all that I can manage, but at least I'm heading in the right direction.

- CHAPTER FOURTEEN -
Shoots of Recovery

Yes, the physical rehab is exhausting but my mind is active and my speech starting to return. Why, there's even some level of timbre evident in my voice. Now if I can just find a sympathetic patient with some of his wits about him, I might even contribute a bit to a proper conversation.

Ian is 44 years old, on his second marriage with two young children, and suffering from a congenital heart problem he shares with his three brothers. He accepts the deck of cards life has dealt him, finding aces and kings where others only see the two of clubs. Once in the army, he served abroad before returning to set up his own business which thrived, until one day, quite unannounced, he fell over: the first sign of the heart problem that was to dog him for years to come.

He seems to take pleasure from talking to me in his broad Scottish brogue. I am an eager listener. He explains how he lost the business, the marriage, the first wife and the fancy motorcar when his health gave way. He believes he's stronger for the experience, displaying an inner warmth and calm that belies the parlous state of the left side of his frame. When on active military duty he had spent many hours in the company of the Gurkhas, refreshed by their attitude to possessions and the pursuit of material things. One particular orderly had impressed him when outlining his plans to buy a scooter. The Gurkha was saving money as fast as he could to buy this vehicle. But the transport wasn't for him. Even though he was buying it, he didn't need to own it. It was his gift to his village high up in the mountains.

The story refreshes me too. It sets me thinking about the chase for the Yankee dollar and suddenly I become very conscious of the profit and loss account that is our life. If my own illness proves anything it's that we should be very careful how we spend whatever years we have. People can tell you but it takes a loss to comprehend value. Do not waste a moment. Time is such a precious resource and, of course, the only certainty in life is a reasonable probability.

Ian passes me an Everton toffee. It looks so appealing in its black and white livery, but that toffee spends the night on the table next to my bed in its clear wrapper. The following day he notices it's untouched and asks why, before realising I can't use my hands to get the wrapper off, let alone put the sweet in my mouth. We giggle at the absurdity of this scrimmage.

The following day he goes back home, the hospital having said there's nothing more they can do for him except wait for the next downturn in his health. What a way to pass the days, waiting for the next relapse. His parting gift to me is another mint. As he hands it over he tells me, "You'll know when you are getting better because you'll be able to eat that sweet without any help." His departure leaves me feeling introspective.

Even though I still can't project my voice very far I can at least make myself understood. Every day the strength of my breathing is measured on a puff machine to assess how much air I can exhale. The pitch is still soft and rather feminine and I favour short sentences lest I run out of steam midway. It's a perfect time to start articulating my thoughts more clearly. After six months I've reached the stage where I want answers to many questions about my prospects and the future.

The matter which doesn't rest easy with me is the sense of injustice. I don't have a foolish diet, I've never smoked cigarettes, I drink alcohol occasionally but rarely to excess and the closest I've ever come to taking drugs is a Fisherman's Friend. I've been very fortunate to avoid hospitals, save for the birth of my children, for most of my adult life. Admittedly middle age has crept up on me. You can tell when the hair from your nostrils grows faster than that on your head, and your eyebrows, left unchecked, start to give the old Labour Chancellor, Denis Healey, a run for his money.

Research into GBS is adamant the illness is not stress-related, yet I'd started to suffer compromises to my condition over the immediately preceding years, suggesting stress was a factor. I don't believe in stress. I think it's one of those 1990's expressions which have carried over into the new millennium, but which should have been permanently consigned to a dusty library shelf – a bit like crop circles, crystals, the word *holistic* and Chris de Burgh.

Maybe I should have studied my tea leaves more carefully. The omens have been harbingering away if only I'd noticed them. The more I think about it. the more I realise the last few years have been relatively poor ones in terms of my physical condition. However, like most men who refuse to read a map when they desperately need directions, I've failed to spot the signs, far less interpret them and do anything about it.

Last summer an outrageously gifted trompe l'oeil artist – he could paint any flat surface and kid you it was 3D – had taken hold of my hand and studied my palm. He began to stumble over his words, he'd bad news and needed to compose himself. "I've got trouble with your life line," he said. "It just sort of stops over here and then starts again over there, almost as though you have two lives. I won't go on if this is upsetting you."

"Geez, you old fraud," I'd said. "Just get on with it." He swallowed and proceeded to tell me things about my life history he couldn't possibly have known, before warning me that my second life line started up again after a big gap: a schism of epic proportions. He told me to learn from the past and hoped I wasn't about to have a dreadful accident.

I've thought no more of that conversation. Until now.

So what can history teach me? Well, there's big Willie for a kick off. Willie John McBride was arguably one of the most ferocious and feared rugby players the British Isles has ever exported on a Lions tour. But, when asked to describe his most difficult opponent, he cited his gallbladder. The pain prior to its removal was the most malicious he'd ever experienced. This we had in common. Three years ago I too felt that red hot poker stabbing away inside my stomach, followed by sweet release when a skilled surgeon whipped out the offending gallstones.

When I'd woken from the general anaesthetic, my children showed me the resultant trophy: two gallstones the size of liar dice in a specimen jar. Hard and pitted like golf balls, they glared at me, defiant to the last. My elder boy planned to exhibit them to his classmates, so away they flew to be viewed by an audience of schoolboys before returning home via a silver specialist who presented me with a fine pair of cufflinks, trapping the gall inside two tiny metal casings. Revenge was indeed a dish best served cold.

Evidently that operation had traumatised my system. It meant – if I had a family history of psoriasis – that there was now a 50-50 chance of the disease hitting my skin six months later. I did, and, right on cue, my flesh started to bubble and burst. Red and angry, it came aboard two by two, particularly around the back of my elbows, the side of my calves and the knees. Pungent smells abounded as all sorts of potions, remedies and creams were applied to little avail over the ensuing months.

It was time for the UVB light treatment, ridiculously paid for by my private health insurance but administered by the NHS. It's available on the state but you'll have to wait for months. The nurse instructed me to disrobe behind the screen and put on some goggles. "Now stand inside that cabinet over there containing the vertical light tubes," she said. "When I close it and turn the light on, lift up your left knee and right elbow to point at the light source, and then alternate."

"Let me get this straight," I replied. "You want me stark naked wearing a pair of goggles inside an upright coffin doing a Morris dance?"

"Yes, that about sums it up," she said. "Oh, just one other thing. We recommend you protect your genitalia."

"Pray tell me, how in all its infinite wisdom, does the NHS propose to protect my genitals for me?"

"We recommend a black sock."

My skin cleared up in no time at all. I really can't decide whether it was down to the light therapy or my stress-relieving guffaws each time I put that sock on. Large, of course!

If you're a gambling man you'll appreciate the odds. Fifty-fifty seems pretty fair if you're placing even money, but a 1-in-14 chance of the psoriasis then triggering psoriatic arthritis would be backing a rank outsider. Yet, sure enough, it romped home about three months later. Cue pins and needles in my index fingers and thumbs, lack of grip and oblique sensations, together with a swelling in my right knee, requiring regular draining.

Now gambling with money is one thing but gambling with your health? That wasn't something I wanted to do. And I hadn't reckoned on my personal bookmaker deciding to raise the stakes still further with his very own GBS accumulator. This time the odds were even more spectacular: 100,000 to one. Who needs the lottery? The tingling in my fingertips, which arrived with the arthritis, was a mere aperitif to the virulent later assault on my nerve endings, which rapidly intensified as my immune system started to crash out of control.

The last few years had offered an insight into the perils of ill health. Nothing more. I had not become used to being under the weather. Now, for the first time in my life, I've met my match. This is the point where I've literally run out of steam, leaving me inert and grateful for anything which reminds my tired frame of movement and activity. I will never dismiss my health, underestimate the importance of diet or postpone exercise again. The lesson has been well and truly learnt, here in my new necropolitic home where the walls are made of perdition, the roof smells so fusty and the windows offer so mawkish a view.

4

How to Win Friends
and Influence People

A Solitary Confinement

CHAPTER FIFTEEN

How to Win Friends and Influence People

Behind the paid workforce there's an army of unpaid volunteers. Known as The Friends of the Hospital, they frequently give up time to serve in the coffee shops, man the mobile library and even bring their pet dogs round for companionship.

Each morning around 11 o'clock one of these volunteers comes to dish out the tea from the three-wheeled trolley (it used to have four, until one broke off). The faces become familiar, as does my response: a beaker of tea with a straw please. Generally the volunteers have their favourite days. So do I. I long for Tuesdays. This is the day I get my digestive biscuits and cup of char from the 'Titled Tea Lady'. Lady Farquhar was obviously a stunner in her day and could tell me my 'head was on fire' and still make me smile, so serene is her countenance. Always immaculate and blessed with a still beautiful face, she makes a fabulous brew and dishes out the biccies with élan. Sometimes I even get a piece of cherry cake.

She invites me to come and visit her little garden when I'm finally released from hospital – the most amatory thing to happen to me since being admitted. I'm transported into a DH Lawrence novel where I'm going into the fields to bring back the harvest, courtesy of the passionate bit in *The Rainbow*. Or can I be Mr Darcy, just for a while, as steam rises from my open shirt and breeches after swimming across the lake? Hoping for a little frisson with a 68-year-old, albeit very well-groomed, pensioner may not be your idea of romantic idealism. But it certainly makes the chocolate bourbons taste a bit spicier. My feelings will, I'm sure, remain unrequited, but she has lovely ankles and her idea of a little garden is 40 acres. Suzi knowingly approves of the weekly twinkle in my eye.

She's far from my only uplifting visitor. There's John Isherwood. As schoolboys the rotund asthmatic and I were inseparable, always sitting next to each other in class, always getting into mischief and always sticking pencils into each other's ears. You might know the sketch where a schoolmaster walks into a classroom and the boys try to stifle their giggles as, in slow motion, a bucket full of water, propped over the half-open door, crashes on to his head soaking him down to his shoes? A scene that's all the funnier because the teacher can't see the humorous side. Well, John's attitude to school was like that – and he never got caught.

I did, however. In John's company I'd always snatch defeat from the jaws of victory: Stan Laurel to his Oliver Hardy. And now here he is at my bedside, making me feel nervous. What possible reckless skulduggery can a horizontal paralytic and a by now very eminent barrister get up to in a hospital? John sees it as his duty to visit me regularly, abuse my fragile confidence and barrel me out of the ward in a wheelchair. He regales me with side-splitting stories, drinks my squash and eats my grapes, ignoring my cries of pain and anyone foolish enough to get in our way. I love him for it.

Another old school friend turns up to see me in hospital by accident. His life has crossed the Rubicon of public consumption since the last time we met, 32 years ago, at the first showing of *Papillon* with Dustin Hoffman and Steve McQueen. I've kept abreast of his medical career, principally by sitting next to the Financial Times' food writer who, it transpired, suffered from Crohn's disease. A rotting of the stomach is hardly conducive to writing about food, but it was how he'd met my old mucker, Dr Andrew Wakefield, who'd spent many years trying to decipher what was going on inside his and other people's bellies.

He'd gained global notoriety after publishing his views on the link between triple vaccines and autism. Vilified by British health professionals, he'd had to move to Austin in Texas to earn a living. He remains firmly in the public eye through the many media reports chronicling his perceived shortcomings as the row over MMR rages. That doesn't stop him being my mate, though, or his friendship with the desperate chap two beds away from me. Formerly the life and soul of every party, Gerry has suffered a massive stroke and is unable to speak, consume food by mouth or see very well. He has many, many friends, all hearty folk who stay for minutes, but no family to stay for hours. Most of the time he cuts a particularly lonely figure. His ability to communicate is as reduced as his number of opportunities to talk to true friends – or his chances of recovery.

Dr Andy implores me to take good care of Gerry. I attempt to do so but with limited success, except when we can find a willing interpreter to translate our attempts at messages. None of his friends stay for long, finding conversation as difficult with him as I do. In truth they've only been his friends when he was buying the last drinks at the bar.

By contrast, I'm amazed and shocked by the number of my visitors; I'm almost embarrassed. Some I've barely known for a few weeks, others I've known since childhood. Seeing a couple of school chums would match my expectations. Instead, my former headmaster, best pal, next best pal – all the way from Australia – and more next best pals in descending order, turn up on the ward. There are men I was once form prefect to, the games master and the Chairman of the Board of Governors, along with the Chairman of the Old Boys Association and countless others, all making pilgrimages to my bedside. Then come the college buddies, work colleagues and business associates, not forgetting my neighbours, aunts, uncles, nephews and past employees, intermingling with friends from America, Wales, Scotland, Ireland, and France. They even turn up from Essex, but don't worry, it's only the one from that county.

Some 15 years previously a school contemporary had been struck down by an illness from the Guillain-Barré family. Known as CIDP it paralysed Roger down his right-hand side in a way which confused the local health authorities. Far rarer than GBS, it was beyond the scope of the regional team, so off he went to London for plasma exchange. Although he made some good level of recovery, his decline was not arrested in time for him to fully bounce back.

Today Roger breezes into the ward armed with a bottle of Guinness and a wide smile. Introducing himself as "your friendly neighbourhood cripple" he begins to set out in painstaking detail the many trials and tribulations that hit him. Since the illness had first taken hold, his marriage and business had fallen to bits, before he struck rock bottom with depression. An engineer by vocation he adapted to his new-found status, embracing life with his remaining active hand. He fought off the depression, and, having accepted he'd never fully shake off the ravages of the CIDP, nursed his children through school and on to Oxbridge. He'd opened his own garage, met a new girlfriend and made light of his disability. Never one to court pity, Roger's lack of regret and deflection of sadness provides a great tonic. If he can get through such a seismic attack on a similar level to the one I've experienced, then I've really no excuse to rest on my laurels.

Should you ever have the misfortune to be in the trenches fighting an old-fashioned war, Roger is the one bloke you want alongside. Not to fight the enemy – he'd be as much use as a chocolate fireguard – but to proffer courage, physical support with his left hand and car maintenance tips, or perhaps bizarre facts about the mortality rates of travelling circus clowns in Venezuela. His whimsical take on life would gladden the soul and help you pass the time admirably. Crucially you'd never need to mention the enemy.

It isn't just friends though. Or creditors. Even my bank manager tries to drop by. I've just offered the opinion that GBS is an illness I wouldn't wish upon my worst enemy when – at that very moment – a missive arrives from the very man himself, offering me great sympathy. Apparently he's contacted my office offering to come and see me, and, with deftness of thought, they've suggested a card will suffice. They didn't want his visit to kill me off completely.

Of course, rumours of my Huckleberry death have circulated, but these are greatly exaggerated. In the case of young Daniel, it must be said, no such exaggeration is necessary. He is brought into the ward so comatose it's difficult to tell whether he's dead or alive. A year to the day his best pal had been killed by meningitis he'd been hit by the same illness. And hit hard too.

The pace of his decline has been breathtaking. One moment he was enjoying life to the full, the next he's battling for his existence in intensive care. He lies in a coma for three days before drifting in and out of consciousness. In addition to paralysing his arms and legs, it has affected his eyesight. He puts on a brave face for his doting family who show vigilant and constant support then burst into floods of tears as soon as they leave. Amidst the many words of encouragement he knows his chance of recovering his sight is slim in the extreme. He can hear all the words of praise from fellow patients in the ward but it's weeks before he can put faces to the voices. At the age of 24 he had once believed his world would include oysters, now the pearls were gone and life was just a swine.

His bedside is buried under an avalanche of unsuitable food. He could sponsor *Coronation Street* with the amount of chocolate in his possession and, unsurprisingly, is putting on weight while the rest of us lose pounds for fun. Every day his friends and family visit in relentless waves, washing over his bedside, regaling him with the same ubiquitous welcome: "All right?" How I long for a 'Hello', 'How are you?' or even a 'Hiya', just to break the monotony. Perhaps if the use of 'all right' could receive greater inflection or some variation in semantic emphasis I'd not object so strongly to the demonstrable lack of imagination. Yet Daniel is making a sterling recovery due in large part to the warmth and union of his family. In fact he starts to improve so much on a daily basis that he seems to be in competition with his immediate neighbour Bill.

At the age of 64 young William had taken a marginally early retirement and just embarked on a cruise with his wife when he experienced the first brain aneurysm. He was airlifted straight to the hospital where it's clear to all that he's in a very distressed state. Stuffed full of morphine he's hallucinating wildly. Yet, after four days, he starts to show definite signs of improvement. From an unequal start he and Daniel are now competing head-to-head to see who can make the most dramatic recovery. No sooner does one demonstrate he can walk down the corridor with the Zimmer frame than the other discards the frame and graduates to sticks. Even though Daniel still struggles to see, he's determined to make his cry for freedom a vigorous one.

I become very fond of them both. After all, I'm their audience. I've spent months as a spectator of life unable to participate in any meaningful way. Observation has become my speciality. It's the one thing I can do really well. The world's still spinning round outside and I've no choice but to become busy doing nothing. It reminds me of a line I once performed on stage in strictly amateur theatre: "Players sir! I look upon them as no better than creatures set on tables and joint stools to make faces and produce laughter, like dancing dogs."

Armed with this medieval quote I set off each day – almost always with the indefatigable Suzi – to circumnavigate the globe, or at least the canteen or The

Friends of the Hospital Coffee Shop with its fuchsia pink-liveried majesty, in search of a suitable table. Seeking out hidden treasures like a stolen slurp of tea from a china cup and a nibble on a digestive tiffin, I watch the unwashed, the unwell and the unwilling do their dog dances on tables and stools.

Observing other people doing things denied to me is a strange sensation. When you're able-bodied, tasks like climbing stairs, walking or cutting up your own food do not register as liberating pastimes. To me they appear so pleasurable, so divine. What a thrill it must be to be able to take part in life, be active, perform tasks without having to summon the stamina – or someone else to do it for you.

My horizons stretch to getting into a wheelchair to taste the sunshine and watch these different types of theatre. Still kidnapped inside my own body, it's a genuine treat to be taken for a push in a wheelchair, and the fact I can sit upright for a period of time is terrific progress in itself. More drama comes from trips to the duck pond, the hospital newsagent and, best of all, sitting under the auburn chestnut trees watching the sun go down over the village green as dappled light picks out ebony swallows darting through the dusk and white cotton clouds soaring over an azure sky.

For a less serene piece of stagecraft, never to be repeated but scored in my mind's eye forever, I can thank my friends Nick and Ali. They take me to see their son, young copper-haired Calum, who's attending his very first cricket school. He's never played before and competitive dad is determined his son will one day open the innings for England. Marching to the crease, brandishing his bat the wrong way round, Calum doesn't make the most auspicious start. He misses the first three deliveries. At best his father's smile can be described as rueful.

The exhortation "Just hit it, lad" certainly galvanises the seven-year-old. He promptly sets off, both arms outstretched like wings, bearing down on the rest of the field while firing bullets from his imaginary Spitfire. After shooting everybody in his own team and then the opposition, young copper knob sidles over to his perplexed dad who asks the obvious question: "What do you think you were doing?" The answer? A totally disarming "Being an aeroplane, silly."

Back on the ward there's a similar sense of the surreal. I've been in the same bed for so many months that I'm fast approaching veteran status. My good buddy Sundance has been allowed home twice, only to suffer relapses and find himself readmitted. His hopes crest when he's transferred to a specialist unit in Bristol for the relatively innovative Campath treatment. After putting his body through yet more steroids he returns to our ward for the third time and what will be our final period in hospital together.

A few weeks later Daniel returns. He's now walking on one stick with a good measure of sight restored. He's brandishing a copy of his local newspaper in which he has circled a feature on the likelihood of the illness striking him in such a similar way as it did his former best friend. He lays out the paper for us both to read, proud of the honourable mention for Sundance and myself. Evidently our hectoring and cajoling have spurred him on. Typical of the boy, he's always thinking of other people.

Although he and Bill have been released from hospital at the same time, you just know Daniel will not return as a patient while Bill has been allowed home too soon. Sure enough, after a series of giddy spells along with loss of memory and balance, he is promptly readmitted. This time the news is not so encouraging. Further examination and scans reveal a tumour in the back of his brain. The choice is stark. He can risk having it removed in the faint hope of some recovery but with the very real prospect of death during the operation, or carry on for, at best, three more years with the tumour riding shotgun.

After the most tortuous period deliberating over the near impossible choice he chooses the latter. The tears from his wife are hard enough to bear but when Bill himself breaks down there's no choice. You have to join in. Nero himself could not have created more drama in the Colosseum no matter how many lions or Christians were put to the gladiator's sword. There it is again and again staring me in the face, the most vivid pageant with more daily drama than you can possibly imagine or have the stomach for.

These distractions serve a very real purpose: they force me to observe and absorb detail like the finest blotting paper. You see, the background reveals the true being of each man – 'if you don't possess it, that man is transparent'. I'm now stocking up my library and man's behaviour in adversity is becoming my specialist subject.

CHAPTER SIXTEEN

How to Win Friends and Influence People

Apparently we're made stronger by realising the helping hand we need is at the end of our own right arm. Now if I can only make contact with mine. The gym is my playground where reconnecting with disenfranchised body parts is the sport. It's a quiet, clean space with primary colour signage and wide mechanical 'beds' in apple green or russet hues. Curtains offer notional privacy while one patient hides from another and struggles with their task at faltering hand or under tenuous foot. It's always cool and rather calm but with a pervading sense of fun thanks to an optimistic team.

When the physios had first tried to get me to sit on the edge of my bed they'd explained how poor my posture was and that I'd only recover my stability if I sat up in a more upright way. I'm now trying really hard to stretch my torso but impressing no one. They wheel a full-length mirror over, stopping in front of me some ten yards away and I recoil in horror at first sight of what I've become. There it is: incontrovertible evidence I'm now, in my stripped-to-the waist pose, the very picture of Methuselah with Buddha's belly bolted on the front. Everything else is skeleton skinny except for the football stuffed inside my tummy, and a face which has aged 170 years.

I never look in the mirror again. So I've no real understanding of the messages my expression is projecting to others around me. One of the great lessons of life, they say, is that the last thing you learn about yourself is your effect on others. In such a setting how can I effect change when change has so obviously had its effect on me? I'm still wrestling with this period of solitary confinement. Can I get parole for good behaviour? Perhaps transfer to an open prison with more freedom? Or at the very least redecorate my cell? The paint finish on the walls is so last year.

Adamant that I don't want any more visual confirmation of my debilitated state, I concentrate on the bits of my body I can see: the lower arms and hands, legs and feet. I send out regular instructions to them, offer motivational team talks, conduct workshops and whisper sweet nothings. But it's all to little avail. Movement is still so elusive. At best fleeting, at worst defiant, the motion in my limbs has been on walkabout for far too long for the frustration not to surface. I start swearing like a trooper. Billy Connolly's autocue would blanch at the volleys of invective which shoot out at random, apparently beyond my control. I shock myself but this doesn't stop me from blaspheming every time I try to rotate my arms only to see my wrists collapse in abject surrender. It's a pig of a time. It seems like so much effort for so little reward.

Apparently I make some people happy, an odd thing to consider when you're crying so much inside your hollow frame. I don't set out to do this but confess that on the days when I try 'miserableness' I can't really get on with it. So I try being of good cheer instead, in spite of – or more likely because of – the tragic theatre being played out by the most unwitting thespians in their agony and despair.

Yet all the theatre, all the drama, is not enough. I need more than this to fill the void when visitors depart and my tears half form as loved ones and friends turn into the corridor and away into the night air. My answer is to consume information at a rapacious rate. Talking books, CDs and DVDs abound and some evenings I find my entire bed transferred into the television lounge. Incapable of changing channels or adjusting volume, my presence makes it very difficult for anybody else to get into the room. So I lie there alone.

The very first programme to appear is a new Channel Five offering: CSI New York. At the beginning of the series a mad surgeon captures young vulnerable women, plies them with drugs to induce a paralysis called locked-in syndrome (LIS), and leaves them in his basement unable to move or communicate: a veritable living death. Hang on a minute, I don't want to watch this, it's a bit too close to home.

I can't change the channel, cry for help, or get up and walk out. The parallels between GBS and LIS are just too similar. I start sweating, my heartbeat goes berserk, I try to close my eyes but can't silence the actors. Get me out of this room, or better still out of this body, now please. But no, nothing. I'm *locked* in, *locked* on, just plain *locked*.

Then the late shift arrives and looks in on me – exhausted, distraught and breathing heavily. I'm so pleased to see them, so thankful they represent escape. The shock of seeing a programme about a condition so similar to the effects of mine seems obscene in such a sepulchral context. Perhaps I'm not ready for the TV room just yet.

So through the day I try to read newspapers. The logistics are tricky as I can't turn pages or prop a full-size paper on my lap. A typical reading sequence goes column five, then two, before waiting for a nurse to pass to refold the paper so I can study one and three. Usually I can't find column four, but I can find the crossword page – manna from heaven that occupies the brain for some time without having to turn pages. Were I able to fill in the answers it might make me more competent. Can you imagine how difficult it is to complete a crossword while trying to remember your previous answers and their effect on the next clue? Let me tell you it's tough. Very tough.

Pretty soon this isn't enough, however, and the work of Mrs Su Doku takes a grip. I really enjoy the number puzzles, particularly as I have to get other people to fill in the answers for me. Remembering sequences of 15 or so numbers, before hailing some poor unsuspecting visitor to use their pen – while trying to hear what I'm mouthing at them – starts out as a leap of faith. But by practice and sheer cussedness I remove the cobwebs from my brain and the addiction begins in earnest.

It teaches me how concentrating on one particular task can so absorb you that the mind blanks out other troubles. There's no doubt that active distraction can relegate the perception of pain attacks considerably. Teaching my brain to regain control of things again rather than abdicate responsibility is as vital in the recovery process as learning to walk or 'going out for a push'.

Some friends just try too hard to help, however. Desperate to entertain they're keen to add dynamism to your life. They volunteer all sorts of activities which you're not ready for. Witness David T pitching up to take me out to lunch when I've only recently mastered sitting in a wheelchair for half an hour without discomfort.

Forward planning has never been his greatest strength, and checking the restaurant dress code to establish whether pyjamas are an acceptable alternative to jacket and tie hasn't entered his head. Nor has the practical question of how to transport me from the hospital to the middle of town over one and a half miles away. "Where's the taxi?" I enquire, to be told he couldn't get one. So begins the 'going out for a push' expedition. Refusing to accept the incline of the hills – or the fact he's 61 and my wheelchair hasn't passed its latest MOT – we set off about as well prepared as a Richard Branson balloon flight.

To be fair, the early part of the journey goes quite well. Well, about the first hundred yards. Then the cobblestones kick in. This is not my idea of haemorrhoid heaven. By the time we reach the restaurant for lunch they're ready to serve afternoon tea. With much persuasion, however, they deign to serve up bangers and mash. It's delicious.

Indeed my napkin thoroughly enjoys the meal. Dear old David has forgotten I can't feed myself let alone get a glass of Merlot to my mouth. The words party, tea and chimpanzee would be contained in the sentence best describing his valiant efforts to spoon-feed me in the middle of a crowded restaurant in a high-ceilinged, over-chandeliered Georgian pump room complete with Palm Court trio bashing out the waltzes. And then there's the return journey. It feels twice as long and thrice as difficult for him, but not so bad for my bottom because I've secured a leather-bound copy of the wine list to rest my withered buttocks on. When we get back he has to have a lie down on my bed. It's almost nightfall.

Journeys are important, but most take place in my mind. At the beginning most objects of my aspiration involve simple provision. For instance I crave tracing my fingers down the condensation on the outside of the jug into which fresh orange juice, mandarin and passion fruit are squeezed with ice cubes and a sprig of mint. I imagine picking it up and pouring a long, lasting glass of bright sunshine before sipping and savouring it to my heart's content

The fantasy is eventually replaced by transports of delight. It's amazing how many places you can visit in your head without preplanning, booking a flight or worrying about what needs to be dealt with on your return. I picture setting off to the sunniest climes via Fantasia, Avalon and the Falkland Arms at Great Tew for a drop of snuff, a homemade gooseberry and nettle wine for the lady and a pint of Hook Norton – in a straight glass – for me. Or I see myself heading to more exotic places where you can drink rum punch all day and never feel drunk, the offshore breeze is always a gentle zephyr and the turquoise sea so clear you can see coral and exotic fish darting around your feet.

Now cut inland to a balmy river, perched next to a weeping willow, where a coxless pair glide by, disturbing a cormorant or grebe on the plume of a rippling weir. Glance west to an idyllic finale to the perfect day where the sunsets are a brilliant reddish pink, monkeys run wild without bothering you and there isn't a dumped supermarket trolley in sight. Call it Utopia, or Turks and Caicos, or just self-deceit, it doesn't matter. It allows total freedom to travel around the world without visa, typhoid injection or leaving the bedside.

Sometimes the mind's destination is less serene, the escapism more chilling. I've always fancied a visit to Novgorod in northwest Russia, close to St Petersburg. Set just up from its own inland sea and cut in underneath the east of Finland it's one of few ports on a Russian river/coastline which can stay open throughout their supremely harsh winter. The analogy is fairly obvious I suppose: I'm trying to keep my mind open while the rest of my body is frozen over.

Such flights of fancy help to keep tedium at bay. In fact boredom is never an issue. At no stage during my incarceration do I ever feel short of something to occupy my mind. What I do miss, however, is the curious lightness of being: moving a limb automatically, turning freely and without discomfort. Something as simple as crossing your legs appears so sophisticated, so clever. The relative talking happily ten yards away has just rested his right elbow over his left arm and is waving his hand nonchalantly at no one in particular. What a wonderful thing to be able to do, complex in the extreme given all the components that enable such fluidity of movement, yet so simple in the appearance of its execution. I admit it, I'm deeply jealous.

If I'm ever to regain such physical nonchalence, it's going to take time. Serious time. As I first become aware of marginal improvement in my bodily functions I try to measure progress on a daily basis. This doesn't work, principally because the changes are so tiny that it's virtually impossible to distinguish progress over so relatively short a period. So I change currency and start dealing in new units of time. The week becomes my Euro. No looking forward or back more than seven days in either direction. I can calculate the percentages better in weeks. After all, your nerves reconnect no faster than one millimetre per day, and some body parts are more complicated than others so reconnection is slower. Things also take a lot of practice. Nothing returns to you without supreme effort, a setback or two, and repetition. I must perform the activites again and again and again.

5

The Sap Rises

A Solitary Confinement

CHAPTER SEVENTEEN

The Sap Rises

Most mornings I'm woken by the lovely Mary. The first call is around 6.30am, after which I'm prepared for breakfast. My head is heaved forward and pillows rearranged before Weetabix is spooned into my mouth. The tea cools before I sip it while one of the staff sits holding the plastic beaker for me. The only meaningful help I can provide is to tilt my head to one side.

By 7am everyone's fed and ready for a wash. Compared to the rigidity of breakfast service you can be soaped down at any time up to midday. It depends who's in charge of the unit, who's in a good mood and how poorly other patients are. But most importantly, it depends whether Mary is on duty. She makes the work of three members of staff look grossly inefficient when set against her organised and determined care of her men. Although fond of the other sisters she lives in an all-male household with three sons and doesn't like working in the women's ward; apparently "ill men don't whinge as much".

She also understands football's offside rule and can talk with authority about the fortunes, transfers and playing formation of most premiership teams, while possessing meaningful insights into typical girl's talk like whether a 4-5-1 was better than a 4-4-2. I'm intensely proud of Mary; she has a unique ability to mix extreme kindness and sensitivity about people's sensibilities with a no-nonsense, hard-working and efficient method. When she leaves, however, her work is not yet done. One of her grown-up sons has been challenging since birth and although able to hold down a job with limited responsibility, still needs substantial nursing as soon as she gets home. No matter how much on-the-job training any person is given, I can't believe it's possible to be taught the kind of caring skills she possesses.

So far our daily wash has been confined to variations on the classic bed bath. Anything more would involve 20 minutes of two nurses' attention to get me into a hoist, swivel me up and over the bed and drop me into a wheelchair. After months of this work-shy regime, she decides I need hosing down and I'm lowered on to the mobile commode, wrapped in sheets like an extra in *A Christmas Carol* and off to the shower we go. My legs are so weak they slip off the foot-rest and drag along the floor, but once we reach the watering hole, it's a felicitous pleasure to once again feel fresh H_2O, without chlorine, on my body.

It's also time for changing clothes. The haberdashery of habiliments is about to open. In the beginning I'd found it difficult to wear pyjamas all the time because my body temperature was so volatile. Now this has settled down, along with the choice of colours for my attire. This is all very well but the mould needs to be broken once more, if only to help re-educate my thoughts to believe I can be human again. So a range of T-shirts, baggy trousers and loose tops is born. There's no sartorial elegance about this move but it adds an extra level of structure to the day and becomes one of the building blocks to repatriation.

Every day I have at least one session of fulsome exercise and, on most days, an additional session of occupational therapy. It's very easy to confuse physiotherapists with occupational therapists unless you study the respective blue and green uniforms thoroughly. The divide in ethos, though, is easier to spot. The physio team tend to concentrate on getting the bigger muscles moving and dealing with fundamental issues like walking and getting in and out of bed. The occupational therapy crew, meanwhile, focus on turning around positions of disadvantage: how to grip a toothbrush, how to get a shirt on when you only have strength in one arm, how to return the ordinary moments of people's lives back to them.

It's the occupational therapists who teach me how to get a jumper over my head and shoulders unaided as far as I can manage, stretching the boundaries of expectation and result until I master the combination of skills needed. It takes three months just to get my limbs into the right places at the right speed, to get close. I have no concept of grip so improvisation and adaptation are vital.

After seven months the middle of my body has started to recover sensation, not necessarily with strength, and from here the repatriation of the nervous system spreads out in an ever-expanding circle. The fingers and toes form the perimeter at the very back of the queue. Ironically, the pain begins to ameliorate by intensifying in the part of the body about to get better. My shoulders go from a position of no movement, and excruciating pain when put into any new position, to one that's even more painful when touched and very, very cold. Parts of me feel that they've been removed and placed in a deep freeze until a thaw sets in. The pain then finds a new home further down the arm leaving the shoulder to wake up again; and lo and behold the faintest movement appears. The triceps recover relatively quickly in the upper part of my arm, months before any sign of life in my biceps. It's a similar story in the legs between back and front.

Every GBS sufferer is different, however. Three more arrive within a month of each other in the women's and then the men's ward. The fey teenage girl is totally out of it, brimful of anger, depression and despair. Struck from the chest downwards with all facial inflection removed, it's impossible to elicit eye contact let alone conversation. She is, understandably, frightened out of her wits. Still, at least her thumbs work. My thumb on the right hand still hides behind neighbouring fingers, immune to cajoling, pulling and prodding.

The two young guys with GBS overlap. Joe the musician appears first, troubled by aches in his hands and seized up through his trunk. For a musician, losing your finger control is tantamount to disaster but he fights back quickly, returning to work within months. He can play the banjo and write his music again before I'm even able to leave hospital. With a shock of dark brown hair and fulsome beard he could audition for a musical Jesus if the mood takes him but not before he has conquered every Deep Purple record he can find. Joe is cool, garrulous, naughty and jolly all at the same time. By being here he helps me to understand GBS better – and by leaving before me he sets a wicked pace to catch up with.

Nathan has taken a bigger hit and is paralysed from the waist down, save for some freezing in the face muscles. An engaging sort, he keeps cheerful and rebellious. One evening our wheelchairs are eased out of the ward in search of adventure, heading into the main hospital concourse around 8pm to witness a daily ritual that could make time management experts weep.

It takes three men two whole hours to stack tables and chairs from outside the coffee shop and place them to the side of the atrium. One of the team is deputed to operate the floor scrubber and polisher, a mighty, extremely noisy beast. It is, of course, vital to smoke a cigarette through such a ceremony, and in truth, it's this part of the work which devours the greatest attention, time and focus.

If done really thoroughly, the clearing and cleaning could be stretched to a 20-minute job for one man, but by introducing the 'Homage to One's Fag' it's possible to add another hour and 40 minutes. Curiously much of this period is spent outside the building, where the men gather, to pace up and down, often in a figure of eight pirouette. The cigarette is always held on the inside of the hand between thumb and forefinger, and passed from one man to the next like a relay baton. They wear glazed yet intense expressions, determined to extract the maximum satisfaction from their drag, as if it's the last thing they'll ever do on earth. The ritual adds a correct level of worship, devotion, pomp and circumstance into what becomes a compelling ceremony – and sometimes the floor actually looks clean afterwards.

One evening Peter and Jane come to see me replete with picnic basket and a battery of Tupperware. They want to take me out to dinner. So we head for the atrium and spread out our wares on the one table the men are yet to stack away. It's an absurd moment of surreal propriety, laced with a plenitude of over-the-top grub: champagne, gravadlax, crayfish roulade, Stinking Bishop cheese and fine napery. To cap it all a candelabra is produced and candles are lit. You half expect a band of itinerant Peruvian Pan Pipers to appear bashing out *Guantanamera* before passing the hat round.

Conversation starts well but becomes more and more compromised as the floor scrubbing pantechnicon is marched up and down, approaching ever closer. The taste buds are being tickled but the noise is simply too invasive. The solution? The offer of a solicitous packet of cigarettes. The cleaners take off with their treasure, extending the usual performance to a record-shattering two hours and 45 minutes while leaving us in peace.

Quite simply we're having fun: a commodity in such sporadic supply since my admission that I feel quite drunk with unbounded happiness. You can keep tea at the Ritz from now on because I've dined at the most exclusive captain's table. The pendulum is starting to swing – the elixir of life itself is doing me good. Each day's highlights are starting to outweigh their lowlights, not by volume but by effect. Cumulatively there are starting to be more things to look forward to than to dread. The aggregate of all the help, support, visitation and affection I'm receiving is compounding nicely. Like a tree which has endured winter without any sign of life, the shoots of recovery are appearing. Admittedly, they're just in the lower branches at the moment. The highest points of the tree will have to wait, but the sap is definitely rising.

CHAPTER EIGHTEEN

The Sap Rises

Getting set for bed involves a certain routine. I need a series of exercises to be completed on my limbs – a ritual Suzi completes religiously as her last act before setting off home, while occasionally leaving my teeth to the night staff. Changing clothes and teeth brushing are tasks I remain incapable of doing. It's a very strange sensation when someone else enters your mouth with an electric toothbrush and a heaviness of touch guaranteed to make your gums bleed. It shouldn't register as one of Britain's best loved spectator sports yet somehow we manage to make a very real case for issuing tickets and charging for admission.

It's not easy to offer advice to someone cleaning your teeth when your mouth is full of their fingers and your toothbrush – particularly if you can't project your voice. However, when any new protagonist is deputed with responsibility for cleaning my pearlies I always want confirmation they'll only turn the brush on once it's inside my mouth. Failure to do this projects toothpaste across the teeth cleaner, and, on a couple of occasions, covers patients in the beds either side. Some nurses want your advice, others don't, considering my attempts to instruct them patronising. It either makes the person doing the brushing feel cross, or prone to the wobbly chin giggles. The evening performances vary in terms of audience size but the record crowd is seven.

And that gives me the excuse for a joke: How many nurses does it take to clean a patient's teeth? Seven: one to carry out the exercise, one to write the notes and one to supervise, along with one to write the health and safety report, and one to clean up afterwards. Then there's one to initiate the training exercise, one to review performance against government targets and one to share the experience. Of course, if you're counting, you'll realise that makes eight – another reason the NHS finances are in such a mess.

It's all very well having the attention but teeth cleaning becomes even harder when one particular nurse, Sarah, explains she has recently installed a computer at home, and as she's worried about fluctuating electricity supply, has invested in a surge protector. To my simple mind this sounds like a character from a film combining the best and worst of 'Allo 'Allo and Inspector Clouseau. "It is I, Serge!" "Serge who?" "Serge Protecteur, you Fuhl." All pronounced in an absurdly French accent, of course. It isn't that funny but it takes a full half an hour to stop giggling, and three weeks before we can talk about anything else.

It's all rather pertinent. I've actually been trying to improve my French by listening to language refresher courses on CD. I'm also trying to pick up Italian and Spanish phrases by talking to the staff. For some reason the Spanish latch on to me as someone who can help them improve their English and want to know who has the most quintessentially English voice. Naturally I turn to Terry Thomas whose over-the-top depiction of an Englishman transcended his Mersey origins. I waste many useful hours with a gaggle of Spanish staff around me learning to say "You're an absolute shower," either in Catalan or a new tongue, *Madridoise*. The results aren't at all successful but the mirth is reward in itself.

Words, whatever the language – however correct the pronounciation – can be so important. 'Be jubilant my feet' is part of the chorus of the anthem, *John Brown's Body*. I hear this verse over and over in my mind, hoping that repetition might stimulate some signs of life in the lower part of my limbs. Initially it seems of little use as I stagger along a corridor with two physios in tow on a limited promenade. Walking is so tough to relearn. There's so much to coordinate from the roll of the foot and pivot of the ankle to the elevation of the knee; from the reflex in the calf to the stride through the thigh and rake of the spine to maintain balance. It's extraordinarily tiring and relentlessly painful because neither leg matches the ability or pattern of the other, with the strain inevitably taken up by the back whose muscles are awakening from their enforced hibernation.

This is all very well if walking along the seafront at Brighton where the challenge is entirely horizontal. But to regain really meaningful mobility I need to get up and down stairs. So poor are the reflexes in my right leg that I can't even raise my right foot on to a shag pile carpet let alone a full-height step. At the same time the lack of grip in my hands makes holding on to a banister difficult, so the ever-patient physio team grip my forearms and talk gently into my ears like horse whisperers.

And yet it's not hopeless. Far from it. There's a tiny flicker of life down the inside of the left leg – one or two messages are clearly getting through to some of my toes. It's just possible to get this foot on to the step and, with sufficient support on either side, stand while concentrating on motivating my left thigh muscle to elevate me upwards. My right side should be ashamed of the paucity of its contribution, but no matter what level of caution, bullying or encouragement is offered, my dexter and sinister remain disenchanted at the thought of reconciliation.

The expression 'hard yards' aptly describes the amount of effort involved for a relatively paltry return. In fact they're more like hard inches in terms of the physical achievement. There's some cardiovascular involvement – climbing the stairs always gets the heart racing but most of the time the obsession is just getting muscles to remember what to do and how to do it. There's no easy way.

Repetition produces marginal improvement each session, the bar then raising itself in anticipation of achieving slightly more next day. If you're fit and able-bodied it's impossible to picture a direct comparison. All I can do is compare how I feel at the end of each of these sessions with how I remember feeling after a five-mile run in my previous life.

I'm starting to feel my age as much in terms of my lifespan as in terms of the time I've now spent in this hospital. All eight months of it. Some of the senior sisters have become more than just caring, helpful people: a union has grown between key members of the team and Suzi and me. Not only are we part of the furniture, we're becoming the mascots.

We don't age in equal units of time, each year marking exactly 365 days of progress. We age in dollops. I was 28 for an awfully long time before I finally accepted I'd just turned 40 – this, of course, at the age of 47½. So if this is my 50th year will I ever recognise it? Will I collect my £200 as I head straight past Go on my way to the Old Kent Road?

I know I'm much older than I was before the illness – I accept Saga will write to me regularly about Stannah Stairlifts, coach trips to Eastbourne and retirement homes in the Algarve – and that my life will never be the same again. But I'm now in an altogether different world. Who is this new person whose washed-out old body I've taken over like a soft crab sheltering in someone else's shell? Questions bounce around in the head: Do I know you? Do I really know who or what you are? And how exactly were we introduced? Answers begin to form but are never complete. It seems too narcissistic an exercise, too self-indulgent, too complicated and besides… here comes nursey.

After ten years out of nursing, deeming her two daughters sufficiently independent for her to go back to work, Liz has returned to her vocation. She sets about her duties with a *viagral* approach (you know, always ready for action and firm in all the right places). She's knowledgeable and skilled, caring and aware. Within moments of arriving on duty you can taste a sea change in the attitude of the staff around her, a sense of being properly supervised. Her warmth and humour are infectious, while her readiness to give Suzi lifts home at the end of the shift provides hard evidence of her philanthropic nature. She also engages my brain in a way none of the other nurses do. She talks to me as though I'm well again, dismissing the things I still can't do for myself as mere triflings. A real cup-half-full person, she reminds me of how I thought I was in my previous life. More realistically she probably just makes me feel better about the art of being.

- CHAPTER NINETEEN -
The Sap Rises

I nstead of just thinking in weekly units of measurement, one forward one back, certain dates are starting to loom as targets: my father's upcoming 90th birthday in mid-July, followed by a move out of hospital into rehabilitation.

Firstly that very special birthday. With a lot of encouragement from the occupational therapy team and several practice runs I learn how to get in and out of a car from the wheelchair. To begin with I find it impossible to swivel into the car without someone pushing me, can't adjust or fasten my seat belt, and have to plan my bodily functions well in advance to make sure I won't be indisposed on any journey, particularly 10th July — my father's big day.

Having fallen over and broken his hip some two years ago, my father has never really recovered full mobility. On the scorching sunny afternoon of his birthday he and I arrive at the sweet little hotel near Bath, determined to see who can strike the most immobile pose. Both of us require Zimmer frames and can barely stand for any length of time. I've never witnessed him writing a speech out in advance – he has always been consummate in his ability to stand up and talk to an audience with wit and panache. This time, though, he's anxious to thank all those who have not only helped him reach his ripe old year but who have also gone out of their way to assist me.

The day inevitably makes me think of the seven grand old oil paintings in Washington DC's National Art Gallery that depict the different ages of man. Each is equally spellbinding in its detail and imagination. You journey down a stream which broadens and gathers pace in tandem with your increasingly large vessel, until you reach a certain point where the journey starts to slow.

I vividly recall trying to explain to my children why I didn't like their most recent choice of white noise music. As soon as I started the sentence I knew I needed to slip my words into reverse gear. Yet it was too late, the words kept tumbling out. When I heard myself say "personally I prefer something with a bit more melody," I knew I'd become my father. That would be Washington portrait number five.

It's particularly poignant to witness my father now stumbling over his words and repeatedly losing his place in the notes he'd so painstakingly prepared. It's just so unlike him. Perhaps it's just testimony to the decline in his powers at such a grand old age. In the event he reverts to type, abruptly discarding his notes with a peremptory "Oh bugger this" before peeling off a cracking Joan Rivers story which brings the house down.

Two of my father's oldest friends from his time in Malta, where they were on active duty, have made the journey from Suffolk. Agnes is as immaculate as ever while Idwal, her husband, is resplendent in his Prince of Wales suit. Time has caught up with his hearing and sadly he's almost stone deaf.

As the party wears on so the groupings fragment and I find myself in the garden under a baking hot sun, resting in the shade beneath a parasol. Agnes and Idwal come to sit at the table nearby watching some young children playing croquet. The heat is starting to affect everybody and pretty soon they both close their eyes, until, without warning, Agnes falls off her garden chair, hitting the grass with an inelegant thud. Within moments every able-bodied young man is in attendance to winch her back into her seat, settle her down and proffer a reviving cup of tea. My mind flies straight over to Agnes while the rest of me looks on, marooned in the GBS departure lounge. In a Brian Rix farce this would have been deemed quite funny, but the most humorous part is that Idwal sleeps right through the event. To this day he remains blissfully unaware of his wife's travails.

I'm very proud of my father for how he manages to get through the day, and for his enduring choice of friends and companions. I confess I'm also quite proud of myself for managing to be there and not disgrace the family. They're all there: cousins, aunts and uncles, godparents, guardians, and neighbours old and new. There are wives, sons, daughters and photographers – there's even a black Labrador. Boy, am I tired afterwards and, for the first and only time, greatly relieved to get back to my hospital bed.

The splendour of the day seems to clear any last remaining obstacles to the next stage of my repatriation. Our thorough research has discovered there's no better place to recover from neurological illness than a rehabilitation centre in Wimbledon in southwest London. It's a curious fact that for all our investment in private healthcare – unless your surgery choice is elective – the NHS is by far and away the best, and in some cases the only, recourse open to you.

The final few weeks are all concerned with preparing for the big move. The long goodbyes become very long indeed. The balance between rehabilitation and physiotherapy, and a vaguely social world, shift towards the latter. One of the leading sisters, who'd taken especially good care of us throughout my stay, is called 'Scary Sarah'. She's tall, slim and elegant, blessed with the most extraordinary bedside manner. When dealing with critical cases she's able to project tremendous empathy through her voice and body language. To my astonishment she starts to cry when someone else tells her I'll be leaving in a couple of weeks.

Apparently I've been a model patient. My ward has seldom had an inmate stay for so long – one who maintained an upbeat outlook no matter what the adversity. So my acting skills have clearly not deserted me. I've assumed they'd wish to bring out the flags and bunting to celebrate my departure with loud shrieks of delight, an oompah band and a certificate from the head of the hospital saying 'Thank goodness you've gone'. But not a bit of it. Almost every single nurse who has looked after me in the intensive care unit makes a point of coming to visit me before I leave.

Indeed, I lose count of the number of staff, from doctors to the most humble part-time care worker, who take the time and trouble to seek me out and wish me well. They range from Jason Gardner's mum who works as an auxiliary – when not cheering on the 'Bath Bullet' to 60-metre dash victories for Great Britain all over the world – to the student nurse who lent me a book on metaphysics to pass the time more quickly. It's impossible to say goodbye to everybody but I do my best. If you ever despair of human nature, of mankind's selfishness or the moral bankruptcy you observe, then I commend a slice of hospital life to restore the pleasure of absorbing values and beliefs we should never take for granted.

It's hard to describe the sort of bonds you form with the people who care for you. The exchange seems so one-sided. They invest time and effort and work into me while I feel unable to do anything other than take from them. I'm told this is not the case. If it's your job to take care of people, then you get your reward and the return on your emotional investment through the improvement you witness, together with the more subliminal messages of encouragement from your contact with each other.

After Kirsten is promoted to bigger and better things within the stroke patient world, Pam becomes my physio mentor. She's the person who teaches me how to climb the stairs. Very Scottish of voice, she's persistent and perceptive in equal measure, ensuring no matter how much physiotherapy we repeat each day it never feels repetitive. Thanks to Kirsten's training she knows what's required to make the treatment varied and interesting, always getting me to do more than I think I can.

Pam goes on holiday just before I leave so we never have a chance to say goodbye properly. Yet the first document I'll be presented with on arrival at the London rehab centre is her postcard from the Alps wishing me good fortune. She is thanking me for being her patient. That's priceless.

We're heading towards eight months in Bath's RUH. So the reliance on food from outside the hospital has gathered pace. A menu that rotates every three weeks come winter, spring or summer can hold no more hidden delights after so much studious consumption. Suzi conjures up all sorts of meals at different times of day to provide the variety and freshness so cravenly lacking from the standard fare. A Thai green curry here, a seared salmon with pesto breadcrumbs there, salads and fresh fruit to keep away the scurvy, all surrounded by looks of grave suspicion from fellow visitors and patients. I adore every mouthful.

One particular friend brings in delicious risotto in a thermos flask from time to time, while my younger son Charlie introduces me to the delights of the cheapest Indian takeaway in town. Known as Desh, the colouring of their speciality dishes is clearly inspired by Britain's traffic light system: red for mild, yellow for medium and green for go… straight to the loo. To be fair to the staff, they hardly object to our rampant rejection of their best culinary endeavours.

On the penultimate night of my hospital stay, Charlie, my younger son, delivers a Desh special, and Sundance, Suzi and I savour the delights of our Last Supper, with the lovely Amy – one of the indefatigable care assistants – playing wine waiter. One of those plucky souls with an impish face and very pretty smile, she has an unquenchable thirst for hard work. We've managed to smuggle in a nice bottle of Rioja for the evening and the loquacious Amy has blagged a bottle opener. It's a very poignant evening. The end of an era.

Mentally I'm desperate to move on to a new challenge, to the next level of expectation and demand. Yet physically, it's a big ask. My body isn't really ready for independence, but I have to try. In my subconscious I know my time is up. My treatment in this hospital has run its course and, in spite of everyone's best endeavours, I need a different level of physical nourishment to get me better. There's just the small matter of leaving a huge piece of my heart here behind me.

Somewhere, hidden in our deep subconscious, we all have ambitions to leave something memorable behind. After we have departed this world a living epitaph would do nicely. Ideally it should enter mainstream awareness: perhaps a building, work of art, scientific breakthrough or precedent in law which defines moral judgments for centuries to come.

Such thoughts of self-aggrandisement are usually the preserve of madmen and politicians, and the scale of ambition is much reduced on my part. All I want is to select something suitable to thank all the staff for putting up with me for so long that isn't a bouquet of inappropriate flowers or large box of vulgar chocolates.

The solution eventually comes to me after much consultation with the staff. I confess there's no mighty drum roll, cutting of ribbons, or local dignitary to break a bottle of champagne open across a newly launched commode. With a minimum of fuss three new office chairs for the new reception desk are delivered, enabling every member of the team to sit comfortably for at least part of their day. They arrive quite deliberately after I have left. Spike Milligan always wanted the words *I told you I was unwell* written across his tombstone. A friend suggests I should have *Goldilocks and the Three Chairs* emblazoned on mine.

Why such morbid thoughts amidst all these valedictions? Perhaps it's anxiety. Possibly it's a fear of new levels of the unknown. More likely it's the sense of impending loss that drives home the realisation that, after all these months in the same hospital surrounded by very unwell people, most of whom I'll never see again, a reminder has been served.

It's a clear message that the dividing line that allows us to hold on to our mortality is so precious that life should never be about what objects we leave behind. In the end we shall all be judged by how we touched the lives of others: the feelings and emotions we stirred in them. Perhaps our effect is the last thing we learn about ourselves, but that doesn't mean we shouldn't do something with it once we realise what it is. Somewhere, lurking deep inside us all, there's a Good Samaritan waiting to get out.

6

Slow Forward

A Solitary Confinement

CHAPTER TWENTY

Slow Forward

The raid takes place at dawn. Two burly paramedics lay me on a stretcher, hurtle me into the back of an ambulance and whisk me in a straight line for London. The sun comes up over Reading, heralding a brilliant summer's day as we arrow towards the leafy glade that is Wimbledon. Quite unused to walking any distance before, I'm welcomed with the instruction that this is a rehab centre and I should get myself out of the ambulance and into the registration area by myself – precisely the next level of physical demand I need. I'm placed in a room with five other men. It feels as though I'm attending a United Nations conference. The fellow delegates are Mr Kwek Bong Hoo, Mr David Ndoo, Mr Salvatore Pucillini, Mr Bola Adebayo and Mr Jeremy Spector.

The Wolfson Centre is a classic example of the sort of building we're now desperate to tear down. Presumably there's an architect somewhere who is immensely proud of his design, who can drone on about the way the natural stone effect and concrete have weathered together. To my layman's eye it's pug ugly. But it serves its purpose well. There are wide clean corridors and polished seamless floors perfect to push a walking frame along, with all main facilities on one level and lift access to different floors.

I try very hard to walk wherever I can, pushing a Zimmer frame in front of me, remembering to keep my legs flexed rather than stiff from the hip downwards: a cycling without a bicycle technique I've begun to perfect earlier. In my haste to get around, however, I'm sacrificing stability. On the first Saturday I catch the edge of my walking frame on a mat placed by the front door for health and safety reasons. Well, it isn't safe and I don't feel very healthy as I then catch it with my foot and fall with a mighty thump.

Because I still have no powers of control over my arms, I'm unable to break the descent. The back of my head cracks on to the concrete floor and my lights go out. Not only has the fall shaken me but it has sent my nervous system into overdrive. I can't feel my legs or back. Pain shoots through my ankle. My ribs are smarting. I'm frightened.

The very same devil who had danced the jig of delight on my tongue all those months ago when I first collapsed makes a most unwelcome return. The head is king of the body and I'm incredibly grateful my thoughts and conscience have hitherto escaped the battering that stormed the rest of me. Now there are flashing lights, thunderclaps, florid helixes and sirens laying waste to my composure. Perhaps Machiavelli is choreographing the tango, invasively performed by the Antichrist, as my trepidation turns to panic. I'm seeing stars all right, but they're not from a friendly galaxy.

I've become used to a lack of communication with my body but this assault on my nervous system is more personal than that – it's affecting my brain. I can't and don't want to cope with the maelstroms. Suzi is at my side in a trice. But then she starts crying and all the bottled up hysteria of the previous months comes spewing out. We weep uncontrollably. She tries to prop my head up on her arm. She's wearing a little Prada number – a stone-coloured cardigan – that starts to turn a wondrous shade of claret as the back of my head bleeds copiously.

The crash team determine that I should go straight to the casualty department of the local hospital. Now I don't recommend downtown Tooting at the best of times, but 10.30pm on a Saturday in Accident and Emergency is not my idea of Nirvana. I'm the only outpatient not in handcuffs. Everybody else is attached to a policeman, high on drugs, roaring drunk or plain abusive.

There is a certain twisted logic in the suggestion that our current police stations should be transferred to buildings adjacent to the Accident and Emergency departments of all our national hospitals. This may well be the most pragmatic option but what a desperate, sad indictment of our society. I'm not a criminal and object strongly to being lumped together with a posse of felons. Do I want to live in a world where suffering an unfortunate injury places me into an arena so intimidating, so hostile and so alien in its dyspeptic culture? No, I certainly do not. So you'll understand why I'm so keen to leave this battle zone with or without conclusive evidence that my brain is still intact. Please just get me out of here …

After making unnecessary jokes about how easy it is to get blood on to a stone (cardigan), my head is glued together and we drive back to the Wolfson Centre in the dead of night. The sense of relief is palpable. I'm kept under strict surveillance for the next 48 hours. This makes it difficult to sleep as I'm woken on the hour, every hour, to check my blood pressure and pulse. If that was the only interruption perhaps I wouldn't mind, but I have also been moved to a different room to avoid interrupting the United Nations conference delegates at rest.

They have also moved Jeremy into the room, dividing us by a lime green and blue curtain. On the first night I'm vaguely aware of a small amount of activity in the next bed which becomes more and more urgent, noisy and intrusive. I'm absolutely desperate to sleep but 'The Fiddler' had started his concert and is determined to mount a fine performance. As the level of thrashing escalates and the vinegar strokes approach I find myself willing my roommate on to his musical climax.

At last the end is reached. The sighs subside, the bed stops creaking and peace breaks out. Surely I'll now get back to sleep after such a tiring day. But to my horror he starts again. I can't believe it. All sorts of envy about his libido – and jealousy that his hands work and mine don't – are banished. Now I'm just plain cross. I roar at him to behave but might as well be talking to someone from Venus, or on the roof. He simply carries on regardless.

The following day I'm told Jeremy is suffering from memory loss and can't even recall whether his mother is alive. He was once the musical director of a concert hall and can still play the piano beautifully – indeed, he often does on the old Joanna in the canteen. His wife is very concerned for him, understandably, but doesn't feel she can cope with him back at home. She asks what it's like to be in his company and to share a room. No, I don't think about telling her the truth. Instead I proffer some vague blandishments and wish her good luck with her deliberations. I feel so sorry for both of them, not knowing which to pity the most.

CHAPTER TWENTY-ONE

Slow Forward

After the first two days of assessment – to establish precisely what I can't do – the physio team sets out an escalating programme of daily exercise, principally focused on my trunk and legs. Standing with my feet together unsupported is beyond me, so when asked to do this with my eyes closed I fall over. Turning around once in a circle is out of reach, as is walking backwards, getting up from the bed, and, with flexibility in my core almost non-existent, touching my toes.

Responsibility for my arms is abdicated to the occupational therapy team and Sarah, the head of the department, introduces me to quite the most wondrous device I've yet to see in any institution, let alone hospital. I'm about to put the Robin into Heath Robinson. The OB Help Arm, to give it the official title, comprises a series of pulleys, strings and levers suspended from a metal frame which is manoeuvred in over my head. My hands and elbows are then clipped into leather pouches to support my arms. Counterbalanced by weights behind me, I feel – for the first time since my relapse – as though I can move my arms by myself.

You may well have lost the use of part of your body through perhaps a broken leg or dislocated wrist. It's painful, inconvenient and very frustrating. I'm not looking for sympathy but trying to help you understand my sense of total inadequacy. When you lose the arm and hand function completely, on both sides of your body, you need to rethink your approach to everything because 95% of the things you used to do for yourself are now beyond you. That's why this is such an extraordinary moment for me – it marks the very beginning of becoming independent again.

Almost weightless it's possible, although not easy, to raise a hand towards my mouth. The scriptwriters for *Thunderbirds* would be very proud of my impression of Virgil – to all intents and purposes I'm a puppet on several strings. A broad grin takes over my face. I'm just so excited.

As exercise rapidly fatigues the wasted muscles, however, my new motto must be little and often. So back and forth to the Help Arm I go, four or five times every day. Progress isn't quick but then I've stopped expecting any rapid advance. My expectations are built around the weekly measure. By sticking to this rule I know life is at last starting to return to my upper limbs.

The OT department has its very own workshop, replete with workbenches and panoply of tools. By now – three weeks after my arrival – I'm moving around the hospital with a Zimmer, in short staccato bursts, shuffling along with a grating sound which enables anyone to hear me coming from miles away. It means by the time I get to the workshop all equipment is laid out ready and waiting. After half an hour of arm exercise at the workstation, I have half an hour to recover before returning to the workshop to start again.

The approach is to perform simple repetitions including rubbing a block of wood with an abrasive edge over a painter's easel, firstly across my body, then up and down, and finally from side to side. Do each exercise ten times, change hands and repeat. Alternatively I have to grasp different shaped objects buried in a bowl of lentils, lift them out then return them: movements designed to wake the senses of Rip Van Winkle's nerve endings. And all are enabled by suspending my arms from the OB and defying gravity with several tightropes but no safety net.

My walking still isn't strong but I've enough strength to shuffle the Zimmer frame back to my wheelchair standing on the al fresco concrete terrace that serves as paradise for patients who smoke. The terrace, with no redeeming architectural features, isn't remotely attractive to most people. But to me it's as pretty as Audrey Hepburn in a cocktail dress. You see, it faces southwest, attracting sunshine throughout the day.

I've become expert at sunbathing in a wheelchair. This may not seem like the most interesting hobby but my front benefits greatly from a daily dose of vitamin D, while my back remains a familiar pasty white. If you can remember one of the early scenes from *The Graduate* you'll have a good impression of where my mind transports me while splayed out across the wheelchair. By closing my eyes I've taken Dustin Hoffman's languid place as Benjamin lying on a clear plastic lilo in his parents' swimming pool. Refusing to entertain exhortations to get off his back and off to work, he prefers to fritter his time away in the California sunshine, listening to Art Garfunkel harmonising with Paul Simon on their way to Scarborough Fair. This seems like a pretty good place to be, and certainly beats the reality of life without use of your hands.

So I try to spend as much time in the open air as I can. It's possible with the regime, which isn't harsh but is exacting, goal-oriented, and quite clear I'm here for three months and no more. The culture is very different from the Bath hospital, with everything encouraging you to take as much responsibility for your recovery as you can, as soon as you're able. Independence is prized.

The daily curriculum is exact: to be washed and dressed at 7am, at a dining room table for communal breakfast by 8am, off to the first physio session 30 minutes later, lunch at 12.30pm and dinner at 6pm. Every day there's a fixed gym session at 1.30pm including such delights as the exercise bike, parallel bars, stretches and contortions on a bench.

Yet it's the warm-up routine I'll always remember. Our group of about ten sit in a circle on hard metal chairs, each of us suffering from various ailments in our own special way. We're all hopeless at each of the activities, yet the competitive spirit surfaces to such an extent that you can see little personal battles taking place. It might be between the stroke victim in her seventies and the alcohol-induced stroke victim in his forties, both practising how to stand upright from a sitting position. Whatever the condition, each of us is desperate to do one more than their immediate neighbour.

Somehow the determination makes everyone look as if they're Jonny Wilkinson waiting to take a penalty kick for the England rugby team. Just like him we put our hands together in front of us, set our feet wide apart and point our bottoms towards Plymouth. The results are a little less impressive, however. Although the supervisors provide music and workout routines customised for each of us, we still manage to fall off the running machines bursting colostomy bags, or start punching the walls as an epileptic fit sets in. It certainly isn't graceful or truly aerobic – as a trip to Champneys is intended to be – but it's vital for all of us to try, to take part and to 'think well' again.

Anthony is one of the group. A bricklayer by trade and Chelsea fan by obsession, he boasts a shaven head giving him the air of the archetypal unsavoury and aggressive football fan. He suffered a series of seizures over the past 18 months which have caused a stroke down his left side. Pressure has built up on his brain forcing the surgeons to operate on his scalp, opening it up over the top of his head from left ear to right ear, as though usually closed by a zip. How misleading first impressions can sometimes be – Anthony is a really gentle man.

He goes out of his way to help anybody else around him and is for ever opening doors for female patients, proffering chairs in the dining room and offering to run errands for the less mobile. In the exercise sessions he takes it upon himself to ensure a chair is ready for me to sit down on, not just any old chair, mark you, but the only one in the room with arms. I'm easily the worst in the group at standing up unsupported when I start, but, thankfully, become more proficient over time. Graduating to the chair without arms is a singular and most gratifying achievement.

These sessions became the fulcrum of the day. I try to increase the strength and pace of the repetitions to create a cumulative effect. My first attempt to sit on the exercise bike involves three people lifting me on and one staying to ensure I don't fall off. Initially I'm unable to sit on the bike for more than five minutes and ride for half a kilometre, frequently having to stop along the way. But hard work pays off. Close to my departure I will last 25 minutes without a break and cycle 10km. This is not meant to impress – it's not a great achievement in itself – but when you multiply the progress with an equal level of improvement in all other disciplines, it gives some idea of the journey you must take your body on.

Mind you, it takes me a whole day to recover. Many times I just overdo it and pay the price, either by losing my balance through exhaustion and falling over, or becoming too tired to carry on. Learning to pace oneself is part of the discipline. Don't do enough and you'll barely improve. Try too hard and it's all too easy to harm yourself.

For Anthony it's about earning a living. What he needs to be able to do is to hold a brick in his left hand so he can apply the cement with his right. Is that too much to ask from life? His brother brings bricks in for him to practise on. Some days he lays a few, other days are more difficult as the hopelessness of his plight hits him, and tears of frustration overflow. I'll miss Anthony when we go our separate ways.

CHAPTER TWENTY-TWO

Slow Forward

Rather like the two curious black diesel engines from *Thomas the Tank Engine,* two Duncans appear in the hospital at the same time. It's easy to see the difference in personalities: one is dazed and confused, while the other is confusing and crazed. It's important to identify them separately so the new soubriquets of Duncan Disorderly and Duncan Doughnuts arrive, joining up with them like goods vans. Both have suffered strokes down their left sides so their speech is relatively unimpaired and they can feed themselves with one hand.

Disorderly has an impossible triple-barrelled surname. His memory loss is profound, although in his business life he can remember creating a wine museum near Borough Market. He's desperate – and fully believes – that he's going to develop more of these museums around the world and is particularly keen to open one in Beijing. He has psoriasis in his fingernails and is useless at doing up his clothes or shoelaces. His new saturnine demeanour is the antithesis of the urbane and cultured man he has obviously been.

Doughnuts, meanwhile, is funny. A broad Glaswegian with a once brilliant financial mind, he has made and wasted a fortune. The demon drink took a stranglehold preventing him from making any sensible business decisions from lunchtime onwards. Although his memory is distinctly selective his humour has remained razor-sharp. He keeps cracking jokes and always spots the opportunity for a gag. When I exclaim I'd love to see the Wallace and Gromit film *The Curse of the Were-Rabbit* (the northern duo's ludicrously fun take on the werewolf legend), it prompts the following riposte: "We know a story about that don't we, children? I used to be a werewolf, but I'm all right naooooooow." His blood sugar levels are shocking to everybody except him, so staff are deputed to prevent him from sneaking a biscuit or obtaining sugar for his tea. His previous addiction to alcohol has mutated into a fresh addiction to sweetness. The former has nearly killed him. The latter will almost certainly finish the job.

Doughnuts latches on to me at mealtimes. It's important to ensure I sit on his right-hand side as we only have his right hand between us to assist with feeding. The dining room is a communal eating area and spartan in the extreme. The days at the first hospital of being spoonfed at one's bedside (or indeed in bed) are long gone. Everything here is designed to make you try to help yourself and I'm as willing a participant as the OB Help Arm can make me become. I can get to the table and, if the chair isn't too low, sit down to wait for someone to push me in and stick a napkin around my neck. I still need to be fed as I can't take the OB into the dining room, but the return of sensation in my shoulders allows me to nudge plates and cups with the side of my arms.

Over the weeks the team, and Doughnuts, enable me to graduate from total reliance upon them to a curious halfway house. The vanguard of this journey begins with a piece of toast but it's complicated, so listen carefully at the back. The index finger and thumb of my left hand have started to show small signs of movement and I'm able to grasp the edge of my first granary slice and, by rocking my body backwards, to drop my left elbow below the height of the table. This lever system pops my left hand upwards – with the toast pincered in my tenuous grip – enabling me to drop my head over the toast and munch my first piece of marmalade splattered Hovis. Frank Cooper's finest it's not but it tastes like sheer ambrosia to me. Admittedly a lot goes on to the floor and much on to my T-shirt, but there's no mistaking: I've managed to feed myself independently for the first time.

Slicing food with a knife or spearing it with a fork is still way beyond my compass. However, by wrapping handle-enlarging foam grips around a spoon I'm able to grip (or rather rest) cutlery in my hands and, with crude lunges induced by my shoulders, can shovel food around the plate before utilising my newly perfected lever system. It's important to try and raise my arm and hand up to 45 degrees and dive down over the food swiftly. Any steeper angle – or dawdling on my part – and the food is on the floor. It's barbaric, vulgar and grotesque to observe but a vital step in reparation. Polite society will have to wait patiently for my return. If manners are supposed to maketh man then this man is making up his manners as best he can.

For a while people seem quite reluctant to sit next to me. I wonder why? But not for too long as the feeding environment has become an arena in which to experiment with miniscule changes in my dexterity. Almost any food is up for grabs as I explore novel ways of getting it somewhere near my mouth. I draw a line at the custard though. It's radioactive. Bright orange by day, they have to lock it away at dusk as it glows in the dark.

The food is clearly prepared off-site by a centralised cook/chill system, ensuring consistency of standard at the lowest point imaginable and a complete lack of culinary intrigue. Once in a while the chill system breaks down and the two girls retained to finish off the cooking process have to improvise and do some actual cooking. The food they put together is just great: flavoursome, fresh and zestful. In fact it's the exact opposite of the food they spend the rest of their working week dishing out.

The highlight for the cooking team is writing out the menu on a white board with a green felt tip pen. It's also a highlight for me because the girls write down the components of the meal as they come into their head rather than in sequential order. So if you're trying to decide what you want to eat for lunch, you can elect to have peppered chicken casserole with chocolate sauce or lemon tart with garden peas. It's hard to decide whether the greater challenge lies in selecting the food than consuming it, although as my patent pending lever system becomes more sophisticated the odds change.

- CHAPTER TWENTY-THREE -
Slow Forward

A reverse curfew after 4.30pm allows patients to leave the building provided they're back in reasonable time to get to bed. The summer is turning distinctly Indian so most evenings offer a wonderful blend of slowly evaporating heat, lazily meandering cotton wool clouds and long shadows from soft shafts of golden sunlight.

Cannizaro Park on the edge of Wimbledon Common, named after a Sicilian nobleman, is a hidden gem of well-balanced tree selection contrasting starkly with the rest of the scrubby common. Less than five minutes by car from the rehabilitation centre it's easy to find a bench from the many dotted around the perimeter. It's tucked behind a hotel where I meet up with Mike Harvey, the old college chum who has suffered a cocktail of ill health to which the addition of Guillain-Barré has been the last straw. What unites us at this moment isn't the devastation our illnesses have wrought on our, and our partners', lives but the first straw: neither of us can drink without one.

We look like spiders from Mars as we blunder our way out of wheelchairs on to our sticks and frames, before crabbing past normal people to collapse into chairs which have the word 'comfy' writ large on them. I listen to his partner Nicola's fulsome tales of sedulous support for Mike through thin and thin. I feel like a total poltroon by comparison with the brave and relentless work she and Suzi have put in to rescue their men. It takes her words to articulate all that should have been said between Suzi and me, but which has remained unspoken because we're too busy doing the doing bits.

Mike is remarkably upbeat but claims to have retired from his previously helter-skelter working life, ironically running the catering for Hertfordshire's hospitals. We look at each other warily, as though we're mirrors reflecting our souls and inner psyche: typical men unable, or unwilling, to put anything but a superficial sticking plaster on our emotional wounds. It's familiar but disquieting. Two old muckers having a catch up. So many things are left unsaid. There's too much ire in our hearts to enable the initial flummery of conversation to develop into something real, deep and meaningful. Two broken souls simply having a tangent before returning to their parallel shattered lives.

The thickness and variety of the mature trees around the park's perimeter create the clear impression we're deep in the heart of the countryside. Admittedly the planes flying over to Heathrow are a bit of a giveaway, but the wind often drives the noise away so it's still possible to suspend belief. There are acers and elms, mighty oaks, limes and magnificent spreading horse chestnut trees alongside copper beech, London plane and weeping willows without a single leylandii in sight. Cannizaro House has a terrace – the perfect spot from which to view what feels like a very private but capacious garden. Dogs set free from their leads bound and sniff their haphazard route defying their owners every exhortation while kites swivel and perch above the treeline offering dramatic swathes of colour and movement against vivid blue skies.

A sense of bliss enshrouds you each day in Cannizaro, often fleeting, yet to be savoured as you absorb the panorama. Suzi is, as ever, by my side, or pushing me or just being there for me, enabling me to sample life. She transmits her strength of spirit by deed and word, still with her own life on hold and with no chance of earning overtime. I'm not an easy charge. But I am a stylish one. I look resplendent in my wheelchair with a picnic basket upon my withered knees. I know what a dash I'm cutting!

When you're in hospital people expect to see wheelchairs and have no need to hide their surprise. But when you're out in open territory, removed from the safety of the medical environment, you present most adults with a different challenge. Able-bodied people are embarrassed by people in wheelchairs. They don't know how to respond, whether to avoid eye contact, smile engagingly or somehow convey 'I'm sorry for you and know how you must be suffering' in their expression. It takes practice and few of the British public have done much training.

As a *wheelchairee* I decide to take the initiative and avoid people's stares. Unless I'm laughing that is, when I look directly at anybody walking past, knowing how relieved they'll be to see someone who doesn't make them feel self-conscious. Children, however, are quite different – they speak what they see. If they spot you being pushed along the grass they'll invite anyone within hearing distance, including you, to explain, "Why don't his legs work?" The answer, of course, is to ignore the question and attempt to distract the child by engaging him or her in any hopelessly random subject that has just come into your head.

Yet getting out of the building into the world of the well is such a vital part of recovery. It's all too easy to give in to one's new-found status as a victim of circumstance. You can become very self-conscious, frightened to confront the normality of an outside environment and intimidated by your own perception of your inadequacies. In short, being disabled makes you antisocial. Well I'm not having any of this, whether my appearance shocks others or not.

Going to the park is relatively easy. You don't have to sit too close to strangers so it's quite a gentle way to begin readjusting. Restaurants, however, are an altogether different prospect. I set off for my first Sunday lunch in Wimbledon High Street with a friend, Nigel, whom I've known since we were seven, and who has returned from Australia for this very meal. We discuss how the beauty of the Wolfson Centre compares to the view of Sydney's Opera House from his back garden and the dilemma of whether to return his family from Oz.

It's not the only dilemma. There's also how to get my Zimmer frame between tables, where to find a chair of the right height which won't slip on the floor as I try to sit down and push back into it, and the issue of how to hold the menu, unwrap a napkin, lift a glass and twist the pepper mill. These are all enormous new challenges in terms of detail, yet seem mere trifles when set against the task of pretending to be a normal person. You so desperately want to be the same as everyone else there but you are not. You are a bit of a freak show.

7

Stronger Body, Stronger Mind

A Solitary Confinement

CHAPTER TWENTY-FOUR

Stronger Body, Stronger Mind

The glamorous Vera, a good friend of many years' standing, interrupts her international jet-setting lifestyle to search the internet on my behalf. Her detective work is sound and she quickly tracks down the Possum 7210. This mighty beast, perfected over many years of trial and error, is built to handle books and periodicals for people unable to use their hands. It turns pages electrically.

Angled like the top of a lectern it's attached to a stand with an electronic touch pad on top. Once seated in front of it I activate the machine by pressing my chin against the pad. It turns pages back and forwards, sometimes shuffling a couple of pages through at the same time, but that's a minor nuisance. At last I can follow a story and pretty much go at my own pace; Cry Freedom indeed. I keep at it, making minor improvements until, after weeks of practice, I manage to get my left thumb propped over the pad and begin manual operation. My right thumb's still studying for his master's degree in shyness, showing no signs of jealousy that his traditional place in the pecking order of duty has been usurped.

The question is: where to site the thing? It isn't exactly small and discreet. There are two principal lounge spaces in which all the patients are deposited between appointments. The cavernous main room is completely dominated by a six-foot wide television screen in one corner. Well-worn armchairs, none of which match any other, are pressed hard against the four walls, leaving plenty of space for patients in wheelchairs to be carted in and out. It's a desperate space, one in which I feel most uncomfortable.

The television's always on so loudly you can't have a conversation, while the battle for stewardship of the remote control wages constantly. I've never watched daytime TV before and have no desire to repeat the experience. To witness the passion which some inmates show for a programme about 12 men, 11 of whom are gay, trying to fool a quite pretty young American girl into choosing them over the rest of her courtesan suitors, seems quite iniquitous. We're acting out our own soap opera. There seems no need for extra rations.

Next door is an altogether smaller room, known affectionately as Fish Lounge because it boasts a fish tank. Not that there are any signs of fish, just the usual parade of bubbling water, pebbles and miniature ruined castles. There's also a compact television screen, turned on occasionally, and plenty of books and reading material, together with just the right space to park my machinery. By placing the page turner in a corner of Fish Lounge I stake out my territory. On reflection it's quite a hostile act. Not quite on the grand scale of invading Poland, or sending Russian tanks into Czechoslovakia one sunny Wednesday afternoon admittedly, but I'm effectively saying, "This is my study, visitors are welcome by appointment only." As I found in the previous hospital, your status elevates, by and large, according to the length of time you have been in an establishment.

Doughnuts and I compose a poem to mark the occasion of the page turner installation. Quite dreadful in its pacing and use of rhyming couplets, we give up after welding the following tribute to a drop of sherry in the afternoon. It's called Xerex, pronounced Hereth.

XEREX

Perfect palindrome or sweet briar,
Milk, cream, Oloross or Amontillado,
Scoop from the schooner, tongues on fire,
Shipped in casks to Bristol promenado,
De La Frontera, Brunel bound with Harveys,
Loved by old ladies, the navy and the armies,
Bang out of fashion, save for Withnail and I, who matter not a jot,
Is that Romulus or Remus craning to sip a hearty tot?

I know, you're right, it doesn't get better in print. But at least it takes our minds off the reason we're here in the first place.

My very first meal in the dining room had provided conclusive proof of the sadness of our demise. I was invited to sit at a table with a gentleman who did a brilliant impersonation of Martini from the film *One Flew Over the Cuckoo's Nest*. Rotund and short, he had a hairy chest which erupted over his shoulders forming a complete link with the hair behind his head, with no signs of a break at the front of his neck. He was wearing a bib under his chin, not to keep the growth of hair in check but to prevent the food that fell out of his mouth from ruining his shirt.

I tried engaging him in conversation several times and, after my fourth attempt, made him burst into tears. I wasn't being rude or unkind, or asking tough questions about the meaning of life or whether England would have been a nicer place to live without the enclosure act, but the poor man couldn't talk. What a bastard! I must have appeared to be on some kind of cruelty kick but just hadn't realised. He was so frustrated by his inability to talk that all he had left to express his emotion was to cry.

As I left the dining area I passed a wall adorned by watercolour paintings produced by the inmates. You've guessed it. The artist with all the gold stars on his work was the very same man. Known as Kahn, he made me feel very humble. Life seemed to disturb him in unexpected ways and I came to realise that it wasn't just me who made him cry. Everything did.

However, when you're the new boy and just finding your way around, you need to make friends. And quickly. Replenishing lost childhood dreams with Kahn through Friends Reunited didn't seem a likely outcome in the future. So after a while I latch on to Royston. A real south London geezer, Roy's on his fourth marriage and has fathered 15 sons. Not a single girl amongst them. He doesn't like being teased about eating more white meat, or adjusting the way things hang in his boxer shorts, and he isn't taking any jokes about King Herod either. Roy has been in floods. To him a bit of damp spells work. A misplaced downpour mixed with a few missing roof tiles means soggy carpets, insurance claims and lots of mess to clear up – Roy's forte. A bit of water seepage from the first floor into the living room is his wet loss adjusters' dream.

I share a room with Royston and we scratch along just fine. He's what's known as a 'character' but underneath the rough diamond exterior lurks a kind and compassionate fellow who'll make friends with anyone. Royston is the usual sad story of a stroke victim paralysed down his left side. Five years of trying to get his left arm to work independently and remove the splint from his left foot have made little impact. Yet every weekend he plays golf to a level with one arm, wraps Velcro around everything that needs two hands to do up so he can tie shoelaces, trousers and bags with his right hand, and compensates for his tilt to the left by walking with a stick. Having learned new ways to put clothes on by putting himself into them, rather than merely getting half-dressed, he is a triumph of simple mind over matter. Nothing seems to get him down because in his world of positive mental attitude everything is just *laaaaaavly*.

Royston also likes a bit of a fry-up and sets up the breakfast club – for 'gentlemen only' – every Thursday morning. Occasionally some ladies are invited provided they agree to be gentlemen during the meal. Picture, if you will, a group of eight men with two useful arms between them bumping their Zimmer frames, prosthetic legs and sticks into each other, in a galley kitchen. Each jockeys for position to get as far away from the actual cooking as possible. More Daddies Sauce and ketchup ends up on the floor than ever does on the plate. Royston's house speciality is eggs over easy, over easy, over easy as once he starts flipping the eggs he finds it very difficult to stop.

My principal contribution to the first breakfast is to get out of the kitchen and sit down. My school report at this stage would surely be too condemning to show my parents. But somehow my confidence grows and I graduate to the washing-up section of the duty roster. Because I can't pick dishes up I develop a sliding technique to prod them along the work surface and nudge them into the washing-up bowl, stirring the murky fluids around with a shoulder-induced twirl of my fairy brush.

Perhaps it's the water that's helping me regain this misplaced confidence. It certainly helped me before, allowing me to rediscover freedom of movement in the RUH pool. By comparison the hydrotherapy centre in the Wolfson is much smaller, although it has no invading coffee mornings to get in the way. The physio team here take turns to look after me, although Anna, the head girl in charge of my case, proves a constant touchstone throughout my stay.

I don't know why I first decide to lie on my back, and set off with a reverse butterfly stroke – probably instinct – and I doubt I'll represent my country in the new discipline, but the level of freedom it offers is immense. Arching the arms to the side, then straightening them up over my head before pulling them down again through the water is wonderfully liberating and, if you're in a wistful mood, has a certain 'Don Quixote's Windmills' charm.

All my time in the water feels as though it's stolen: it suspends belief and reality. As soon as I get out I find it impossible to replicate anything like the amount of movement I've just enjoyed in the pool. One morning Fiona, a fiercely fit and desperately hearty physio, takes my hydrotherapy session. She's very determined, cajoling me into a whole raft of new movements.

At one point, as she tries to make me jump backwards in a somersault and to bring my feet up above the water level, she demands greater levels of exertion: "Go on, get it up there, make me happy. Go on, get it right up there now. You can do it… that's it. Yes, yes, yes!" I ask her if she has ever thought of becoming a script writer for a porno movie. The joke dies as soon as I crack it but I don't think she ever realises what she has just said. It's little surprise, as her focus is solely on my wellbeing. To get me able-bodied again is a target that unites us and I'm hugely indebted to the practised skills, methods and can-do culture she and her colleagues relentlessly supply.

Other friends are desperate to help. In an effort to give Suzi some respite from providing daily care, a number of buddies volunteer to look after me. Many of her best pals support her as much as they so kindly nurture me. On one particularly delightful Saturday an old college girlfriend of mine called T, who lives nearby, collects me from the Wolfson, placing wheelchair and Zimmer frame into the boot of her car, and whisks me away to the delights of Richmond Park.

By this stage in my recovery I can manage short distances pushing the frame out in front of me but find it difficult on uneven terrain. So we set off in the wheelchair, dodging deer, cyclists, joggers and golfers looking for miss-hit balls. There are black clouds in all directions save for the spot of blue sky directly over our heads, and we enjoy a totally unfettered time as the shaft of sunlight leads our march across the park and back again. We rest on a small pedestrian bridge to play Poohsticks, or rather T throws the twigs into the water and tells me which one is mine. When set against the problems that my fellow patients have to endure, such opportunities to recapture one's zest for life make me feel like a very rich man indeed.

No one can say I'm alone in my solitary confinement. There are so many offers of help, from the support of my family to work colleagues, from new friends to old allies with whom bonds were forged decades before. In this, the hottest of furnaces in which to test affections, extra layers of gratitude and thanks are tempered and shaped. The strength of ties previously untroubled has well and truly been stretched. For this I'm so much more fortunate than many. There are other cases around me that are so harrowing I feel blessed to be who I am, in spite of my infirmity. So fast am I running out of Brownie points to award those who have helped, as Suzi has qualified for 99% of the quota, that I decide to switch to Brownie point 'futures' to loosen up the market.

- CHAPTER TWENTY-FIVE -
Stronger Body, Stronger Mind

Unlike the Bath hospital the Wolfson Centre admits patients with a much wider set of reasons for their infirmity. Winston, a powerful and athletic Caribbean man, had been set for a routine operation when the administration of the anaesthetic went wrong, leaving him substantially paralysed in parts of his body and unable to stop shaking everywhere else. He constantly tries to talk yet can't articulate anything that closely resembles words, or adjust the volume of his mutterings. You become hardened to such intrusions when you sink back into your private world but Winston's case is desperate. His wife and daughters come every day to administer food and help, displaying such fortitude and strength of character in the face of the horrifying adversity Winston presents them with.

Another of the patients looks like Charles Manson. With long grey hair, sallow skin and a tattoo on every knuckle and limb he's an intimidating sight. Jack is confined to a wheelchair after being attacked in a pub by a madman with an axe and a screwdriver, an assault that punctured his lung and cut through a nerve in his spine. The attacker was arrested the same day after two further assaults which became murders: a drug-fuelled rampage that emasculated or terminated lives indiscriminately. It has left Jack obstreperous and difficult to deal with, needing help yet not wanting it, and with dyspeptic ways that intimidate the staff. No one ever volunteers to look after him. He is trouble.

By comparison with his partner Linda though, he's a pussycat. She's clearly an addict and impossible to have a normal conversation with. Hyper, neurotic, erratic, prone to tears and downright weird, she plainly still loves her man but can't give him the comfort and tenderness he craves – she can't look after herself let alone anyone else. I study Jack's hands and notice the left one has the word 'love' spelt out on the four fingers. On his right hand is the word 'hat'. I make the mistake of asking what happened to the missing 'e'. "Got bored" is his reply. Before long, though, a smile slowly breaks out across his face and very quietly he whispers, "Besides, I'm very partial to a bit of e."

His history and fate set my mind wondering. Many years previously I studied a day release course at college in Dundee. For some bizarre reason I thought it would help to become a member of what was then called the Institute of Personnel Management. The first year covered sociology, psychology and statistics, and on Monday afternoons a disparate band of students united to broaden their minds. The subject matter gave 'paint staying wet' a run for its money in the dullness derby, but we fellas kept going because of some very soft cashmere. Outlined by her ivory white jumper, Ali's pneumatic breasts enjoyed cult status, holding the male students' gaze for entire lectures.

Occasionally she'd speak and we were all torn because the lilt of her Kirkcaldy tongue, urchin haircut and the retroussé nose all added an extra lush to her lusciousness. Each component was worthy of its own fan club, but the eyes could do nothing to stop man's appalling ability to compartmentalise women, and soon the breasts would take centre stage again. What a handicap.

I sat next to the charming Martin Cleghorn who was attending the course because his father told him to, and who was in total awe of the cashmere queen. He worked in cloth manufacturing in Dundee and hoped one day to succeed his father in owning the family business. However, Martin had not covered himself in glory when first deputed to the personnel department, failing to follow company procedures to validate job applications. Not only had he employed a 60-year-old triple axe murderer, who brought shame and dishonour on his father's company by committing the crimes during working hours, but unwittingly Martin had also employed the man's son who went on to complete his own triple axe murders. Even worse, these were during working hours too.

If you're going to commit triple axe murders – somehow triple screwdriver murders doesn't have the same ring to it – you should at least have the decency to do it in your time off. Martin and I kept in contact for many years and he always signed postcards 'Yours as ever, Jute the Obscure'.

I really can't work out whether Jack would be better off becoming the third murder victim of his axe and screwdriver brandishing assailant, or eking out this existence confined to a wheelchair: cast adrift in a permanently fetid orbit. The conundrum troubles me for days before I realise Jack would have continued to abuse his metabolism by consuming every substance around, flagrantly challenging his body to process alien drugs and support his wellbeing as if he was enjoying a healthy lifestyle and balanced diet. There would have been no turning back.

On the day when the frightening Linda isn't present, his 17-year-old son visits him dressed almost exactly in the style of Donovan, the eponymous 1960s folk singer. I study the interaction between them. The son has become the guardian of his own parent. How much and how quickly the boy must have had to grow up to fulfil the role his father is no longer capable of. How much the father now relies upon the son, in a complete juxtaposition of his former stance.

Perhaps the Wolfson, which runs on hugely proficient lines, has come to rely upon the work of one man as much as Jack does on his son. Its Principal, Dr A, a character worthy of Peter Sellers – imagine a combination of his Dr Strangelove and his hapless Indian actor in *The Party* – is a lovely man, much admired by all of his staff and adored by those patients able to recognise his extraordinary powers of humanity. Apparently without social life or family to comfort him away from work, he never seems to leave the building and has the uncanny knack of entering your room unannounced at precisely the point when his presence is needed most. Mr A rarely speaks directly to you as he's painfully shy, preferring to talk to an area high up on the wall over either one of your shoulders. But while eye contact's rare he compensates with a dry humour and abundance of compassion.

At first glance you might suspect him of being an incidental figure floating along the stream of life in some misanthropic way, yet this would miss the substance of the man. His encyclopaedic knowledge of all his patients, former staff and current charges, as well as supernatural eyesight for any situation requiring his presence, is extraordinary.

The way staff gravitate towards jobs within the centre demonstrates our tribal instincts are not yet dead. The physio and occupational therapy teams are, without exception, Caucasian, well-educated and middle-class. The catering team are from deepest Africa, desperate to escape military coups and mass slaughter at election time. Irish and Filipino staff tend to do the hands-on care assistant work including making beds, washing patients and pushing wheelchairs. None ever complain or go into a huddle to moan about a colleague. They are all unfailingly cheerful and united, ensuring the very special needs of the patients remain the permanent focus.

Like Khan, Royston and Winston, the patients come from all walks of life and their case histories are endlessly fascinating. Carol, whose flowing Titian hair betrays her Irish heritage, is in her early thirties, blessed with two charming young children and an incredibly patient and supportive husband from New Zealand. Two aneurysms have paralysed her down the left side, forcing her to retire to a wheelchair. The paralysis through her left leg and arm has spread into her face giving her mouth a lopsided smile.

One of the main reasons for her debilitation is the effect of smoking on her arteries, a message that has not reached her conscience. Every opportunity she has to get a cigarette into her mouth she grasps with her one good hand. You can tell that as a schoolchild she was always the cheeky one at the back of the class. She has a wonderful air of mischief, and talking to her makes you feel you're both about to get up to naughty little tricks. The renegade atmosphere she creates is contagious, mixed perhaps with a hint of sedition from *Huckleberry Finn* and a dash of *Catcher in the Rye?*

Carol is starting to go on home visits at weekends to see what facilities social services need to adapt for the time when she finally leaves hospital. At home her husband sensibly doesn't allow her to smoke, provoking fierce arguments. It's desperately sad to see the love between them, yet to witness two people lashing out at the person they care about the most.

It makes me realise how fortunate I've been to get this far through my recovery without losing the emotional plot, or allowing the overwhelming egregious nature of my decline to get the better of me for any meaningful length of time. I couldn't have done this on my own. Thanks to the implacable Suzi we keep our spirits up, stay positive and always find things to celebrate and savour. I have a nice view to look at every time she appears, but Suzi gets the short straw – she has to look at me.

It isn't easy; ebullience isn't a crop routinely harvested in the field next door. The process is too enervating for that. But two events provide a memorable boost to morale. Firstly a couple of friends, Stuart and Tony, bowl down the motorway from Manchester to southwest London. Their raucous sense of humour reduces me to mirth just as the misery gremlins are drawing in. Whilst admiring the top of my head they ask me how the physio is going. I start to bore them rather about the minutiae of my daily exercise regime when they interrupt. "We're not interested in the physio for your body, we mean how's the physio for your hair? Surely you can't go around with a barnet like that without needing someone to exercise it and make it do trunk curls?"

Don't worry, I'll get back at them one day, but their determination to force me to laugh at myself is an ideal tonic – almost as ideal as an escape to the country. Suzi and I have accepted an invitation to a special day out in rural Oxfordshire, a journey of almost 90 minutes each way. By far and away the furthest we've travelled from the hospital, it's a real test of our organisational skills, my bladder and general stamina. As we arrive at the village green, bordered by lime and oak trees, we're welcomed by a lamb roast which has been cooking slowly since breakfast. It looks and smells divine. It's a soporific scene, efficacious in the extreme.

For our delectation a grand spectacle is being performed utilising some white – and some not so white – items of clothing, wickets, bats and balls, together with 30 highly unfit family members including long-lost uncles, nephews and nieces, plus the odd ringer, hired assassin and semi-professional. Normally there are 11 characters per side but this is a day for extraordinary substitution rules enabling everyone to take part no matter whether boy or girl, able or not. The cricket may be a joy to watch, but it really doesn't matter because there are so many other things to soak up while the sun's shimmering heat rises above the tree line.

This is a world I have not seen for the best part of a year: the British countryside in full late summer bloom, looking as capricious and becoming as I ever remember. Blossom frescoes the trees, hedgerows overflow and leather hits willow, while I watch lazy butterflies and listen to the clink of fine bone china tea cups: sights and sounds to remind the senses of the diverse pleasures nature gives us for free, pleasures we too often studiously avoid in our desperate dash to get to work on time, attend meetings, and make things happen.

I behold a full colour 3-D world as if I've just been released from watching black and white television for months on end. Participation still has to wait, of course: what a privilege it must be to walk unaided, to hop, skip and jump, drive a car or butter your own scones. But the day makes me deeply conscious of the fact that I've never once realised how lucky I am to have enjoyed such consistent independence of movement and thought for the last 50 years. How I want it back.

The main event, however, isn't the cricket match. While I settle into a deckchair two young children commandeer my Zimmer frame and turn it into a mobile leisure centre for the entire afternoon. They use it as a climbing frame, run races with it – and through it – creating their very own version of Highland Games. They show remarkable ingenuity. The girl turns herself into a Dalek, carrying it around on her shoulders, and commands her younger brother: "Do as you are told or I will be forced to exterminate." As soon as her back's turned, the boy picks it up, flips it on its side, wheels facing downwards, and pushes it like a wheelbarrow. The window into their world is wide open and unashamedly I stare right in, relishing every moment of their innocent delight.

As the heat starts to evaporate from the day and the sun begins its slow descent, Suzi and I set off back to the Wolfson Centre. Not much is said on the journey. We both know what a special day it has been and that another substantial rung in the ladder has been scaled. I'm not miserable when we get back, just pensive, and suddenly very aware of how institutionalised I've become. Unused to the wideness of the outside world, I've been shut off, incarcerated, hidden, forgotten and squashed by this year of years. Hospital rooms are the norm, not expansive vistas or delicious panoramas. Disabled people are my peer group, not happy adults and children frolicking in the fields. I want my life restored. This mugging has taken it away from me and I'm not going to rest until I find it again.

- CHAPTER TWENTY-SIX -

Stronger Body, Stronger Mind

If cricket seems to be taking centre stage rather often in this tale I make no apologies. For this is the year we regain the Ashes. The year England finally lay to rest the various Australian ghosts which have haunted them since the 1980s. Cricket is also one of the few sports which you can pick up and put down through an entire day as either side's fortunes ebb and flow. The pleasure may only be vicarious but it's definitely visceral, as Freddie Flintoff captures the hearts of many previously uninterested people. The margins are very thin between success and failure, but that doubles the pleasure for this partisan Englishman.

Yet, like most Englishmen, my pedigree is a bit mixed: French Huguenot on one side, Irish and Scots on the other. Indeed, I wasn't actually born in the country. I'm Maltese. George Bernard Shaw once described Malta as Europe's largest unfinished building site and he wasn't far wrong.

Yet Malta possesses one key thing: history. It has shedloads and boatloads of the stuff, most of it based around the two harbours of its capital Valletta. Grand Harbour is the most magnificent cavernous amphitheatre with its honeyed sandstone, turquoise water and *dghajsas* (pronounced dicers), the indigenous craft scurrying around like busy ants. Images of the small multicoloured boats – each painted with an eye to ward off the sea's evil spirits – have remained in my mind since returning to England at the age of three.

Little did I know what a poor exchange this was in terms of weather but the real loss was of my deep-rooted love of these native vessels. In a child's mind these boats had a life of their own where their main job was to keep a watchful eye over the Mediterranean's sardines, mackerel and occasional dolphin – and also to watch over me. We all have our God, I suppose. These inanimate craft provided my first lesson about man's need to worship something.

Religion has woven its way through my recovery in many varied but fleeting ways, beginning on the hospital wards in Bath. A pious father from a Benedictine monastery, who had remained detached from the toils of the real world since the end of the Second World War, proved the most uncharitable companion. This quixotic man had the opportunity to make an impression on all the other unfortunate souls on his ward. Instead, he chose to carry on as though adhering to a monastic vow of silence and spread no Christian kindness by deed or word.

I accept his stroke had debilitated him, causing great hardship, yet he was patently more mobile and able to talk and to give to his newly found brothers-in-arms than anybody else in the adjacent vicinity. To him we did not appear to exist. Perhaps he was offering silent prayer on our behalf but I doubt it. I saw more evidence of Good Samaritan work from hundreds of people around that hospital than I ever saw from Father Donald.

Each Sunday night there was a service in the chapel and volunteers went into every ward to drum up support. I joined them on some evenings and on others just sent my spirit. More regular than my attendance were the visits from Sally, a near neighbour of my father. She came partly because of the personal connection but also in her capacity as a volunteer. She helped the hospital chaplain by making pastoral calls throughout the wards, aiding those souls who were lost, supporting those who were nearly found, and facilitating for those few knocking on heaven's door.

Which begs a question. Is it fair to make peace with your God, whoever he may be, when you're in desperate need? You should ideally cut your deal when the stakes are more evenly balanced. Yet life rarely works like that, as you only know if a vacuum exists in your life at points of high drama or great loss – and few of us have access to God's email address for rapid expressions of repentance.

Certainly, I did witness people turning to the Almighty. Elaine, a very pretty girl from Frome, camped in our ward next to her husband's bed for six nights on the trot. He had been experiencing muscular problems and had fallen down the stairs in their new home. Concerned relatives and friends were allowed to ignore usual visiting hour rules to stay on-site pretty much throughout the day but you never normally saw family around at night, so it was particularly concerning she should need to keep up a 24-hour vigil. The marriage wasn't going well and the tension between this handsome pair was sad to behold. An athletic and powerful man in his early thirties, Mark was overwhelmed by her desire to make things right between them. Deep down he knew her guilt was the motivating factor.

They started to pray together, offering what tearful oblations they could. At nightfall as the lights were softened in the ward, they pulled the curtains around Mark's bed and Elaine laid out an air mattress on the floor. They held hands and spoke at length to their Lord, 'moaning in the gloaming'.

Faith can arrive in many ways. Sometimes it comes along and smacks you in the face, sometimes evangelists impose their religious beliefs upon you, and sometimes God seems to have deserted you. As for me, I was, and at the Wolfson still am, finding it difficult to believe in an afterlife or reincarnation. If I do, I'm unsure whether to return as an insect, the county of Gloucestershire, a piece of wood – or Keith Richards' right hand. I'm unconvinced, not knowing whether I've already died and come back for a second go as a poor impression of myself. I don't feel at peace with my God. We're on speaking terms but not the same wavelength. Truth is I still haven't found the answer to the semi-secular question which has dominated my thoughts for months on end. It isn't a long question, it isn't particularly complicated, it just needs a straight answer. Why?

I'm sure Suzi has pondered it too. Many times. After putting her life on hold for so long, she has at last been persuaded by her girlfriends to take a few days off with them. Such temerity. How dare she go away and be normal? It's heresy, I say, a grand treasonable offence.

They've flown to the French Alps where a swell time is had by all. After relaxing for the first time in months, she returns to England and decides to take a shower before coming back to the hospital. She reaches up for the soap and her left arm flops to her side. She tries again and the arm collapses in the same fashion.

Being the practical person she is, there's a moment or two for composure before calmly moving the left arm around her head again, this time with easy movement. When she gets to my bedside she's upset and tearful. There's clearly something wrong and the nurses and I persuade her to seek help. She is rushed away to be examined.

I visit her next day as she is staying overnight in a nearby hospital, awaiting tests. It's a juxtaposed scene: Suzi making light of things but now the patient, being tended by me in a wheelchair, sequestered into her own first floor room. There's no immediate conclusion. Various theories are proposed, several possible outcomes left open. It's weeks before it's decided she might have had a small stroke or transient ischaemic attack. The pressure is telling on them. And on us.

It isn't just the facts of the matter, it's the injustice. How has my demise triggered such a stress-related response and made that pernicious little question pop up again. Why? Why? Why? It's just not fair. She has worked so hard to prevent me giving up, and maintained such a fantastic serenity and evenness of mood throughout, that I'm far more upset for her than I've ever felt for myself. Here we are in hospital with every conceivable testing aid available and still we can't be sure what has happened or what it might lead to. What lesson is God teaching us now?

I'm unlikely to find out here. Religion doesn't enter the curriculum at the Wolfson. Instead we have *The Archers* every Thursday. For an hour we have poems, recitals, stories and jokes read to us by a character actor who has, for almost 30 years, played the same role of Nigel in the institution that is Radio Four's indomitable incarnation, *The Archers*. Gamely he plays out his thespian role but we're a challenging audience. We never clap or laugh in the right places. We nod off during the punch lines and are incapable of summoning an encore. He's playing sweet music inside my head though and for that I'll always be grateful.

In itself his words are not particularly poignant but his tune is redolent of a bygone era when I'd no fear of my own mortality. In fact, it reminds me of the exact moment when my first puppy dog Holly, aged six weeks, chose to come and live life as a Sheppard, selecting herself from a litter on a farm in that village – the very one in which *The Archers* is set. The actor has provided the catalyst to help my mind fly up and away from the rehab centre and back into a comfort zone of pleasures past. It isn't a sententious interlude he provides but a chance to reconnect with one's beliefs and, dare I say it, for some of us to uncover our faiths.

Yes, faith is here all right, written indelibly in the beliefs of the vexed relatives, volunteer helpers, patients with an ounce of optimism and in the handbooks of the senior staff. When faith slips out of my grasp from time to time, I find it incredibly difficult to cope with the levels of sadness. Sadness that sits like a foggy shroud as it surrounds me amongst my peers and supervisors. How I long for the time when I could take my dog for a walk along a country lane and throw sticks while trying to catch the wind and shoot the breeze – all at the same time.

My body still isn't ready to leave the Wolfson but, just as I found towards the end of my time at the last hospital, I'm starting to feel terribly restless and in need of change. Amongst the more recent new patients are three men and two women who have had operations on their heads. They now have sizeable chunks of their skulls missing. To the experienced hospital worker this isn't surprising but I can't hide the fact I find it harrowing in the extreme. The college report claiming my attitude to one particular subject had 'given rise to grave disquiet' makes perfect sense. My stomach knots each time I look directly at these new fellow inmates and the feeling I experience is undoubtedly one of disquiet that's ever so grave.

One of them, Peter, is a very cheerful soul, diminutive in stature, big of heart and kindness personified. Part of his scalp has been peeled back to remove the offending growth leaving a lunar landscape on top of his head which he mocks, claiming, "You don't need a clear night sky to see the moon anymore."

In some ways I still appear to be facing more of a struggle than Peter. During the gym sessions he's much better at mounting the staircase, except he wears a cyclist's crash helmet lest he slips. By contrast, when it's my turn to scale the 21 steps, I need someone with me at every point, both up and down, and a seat at the top to rest and hold on to so I can turn round.

However, while I can't imagine a life with such limits permanently in place, Peter's head will take years and several operations before it looks anything like normal again. And that's just the prognosis from the outside. Inside his brain Peter's struggling desperately to recover his speech pattern. He keeps the words coming all right but they rush out far too quickly and with woeful enunciation.

It's so difficult for him to make himself understood that the poor man becomes incredibly frustrated. His impression of the opening lines of *Four Weddings and a Funeral* is as foul mouthed as Hugh Grant's early salvo of invective but with too few 'fcuks' and too many 'rollocks' to warrant his replacement. Indeed if one chose to be super critical it sounds more like 'muck, muck and ggollocks' which must provide great comfort to Hugh – his top spot is not in doubt.

The side of Peter's brain which still functions perfectly can't adjust to the loss in translation from one side of his head to the other and concentrating is extremely difficult. Television is all right but reading dreadfully hard work, so I read to him from my electric page-turning library. We race through *The Kite Runner*, delight in the joys of *The Shadow of the Wind* and become rather disillusioned part-way through *The Da Vinci Code*. At the three-quarter way mark, it moves from reasonably paced vivid plot with blockbuster film written through every page into a stodgy mess with a storyline that unravels like a secondhand ball of wool.

Our exclusive book club changes, however, as several patients wheel their chairs in alongside us or flop down into an easy seat to rest their weary false limbs. We have an audience. Doughnuts and Disorderly are regular recruits, as is Keith, a once prolific journalist whose fondness for beer had so unsettled his constitution he'd lost his right leg, while his left side suffered the stroke paralysis so prevalent among fellow inmates.

As our book club grows, the two lounges divide in culture. The larger sitting area remains full of people wrestling for control of the remote buttons to switch TV channels. Meanwhile, in our smaller study, the once erudite and learned atmosphere is fragmenting as the number of attendees rises and banter escalates. Generally I start out reading to others only to be interrupted so often that getting beyond one chapter is a rarity.

I switch from novels to poetry. Thankfully no renditions of Xerex but a bit of John Donne, Roger McGough or Linton Kwesi Johnson, which proves a nice appetiser before a main course of Lord Byron, William Blake or Pam Ayers. But humour isn't a common denominator for all poetry. Great poets often write after bursts of severe depression or exposure to pusillanimous sadness. Our fulminating group can be rendered silent if a particularly poignant line strikes the right cordant note. There is poetry in pity and we are a pitiful and piteous audience.

It may have been pity that first inspired the charitable trust funding on which so many of today's hospitals are based, but there's no doubting its continuing effect. The Wolfson Centre is founded on just such charitable finance, which should ringfence the property for another 50 years. The building is dwarfed by the remains of the vast Atkinson Morley Hospital with its majestic – now archaic – Victorian architecture. The estate has been reviewed by the trust responsible for the hospital's future. After much debate, investigation and studies the obvious conclusion is that the land on which it stands is worth much more if the building is knocked down and converted into housing. Similar decisions have been made all over the country: selling England by the pound. It's a costly mistake we'll rue for generations to come as the national hospital land bank disappears and its property-based reserves perish.

Our bedroom block is surrounded by workmen feverishly laying down the infrastructure to allow former staff houses, operating theatres, canteens, wards and private rooms to be bashed about or torn down. Like an oasis in the middle of the desert our curious rehabilitation centre should remain unbowed for generations to come: an isolated island in a sea of des-res sprawl surrounded by off-plan salesmen, show homes, Bosch cookers and duvet delights.

Although still incarcerated at the Wolfson, I'm becoming much better at being taken out for short distances by car. I'm now getting out and about every day while relearning once simple tasks like pulling the seatbelt across my chest. This involves putting the back of both my hands together on either side of the belt and using my chin to apply the grip when compressed against my shoulder. Adapt and adopt is the new motto.

My bodily functions are displaying pockets of improvement including mobility in my shoulders and relative strength in my triceps. I overcompensate hugely with the bits of me that work to make up for the recalcitrant parts that still don't. Thankfully there's a compounding effect so a marginal amount of additional strength is generated every time I stand up from a wheelchair or sit back down into it.

My shoulders still dominate all upper body expressions of movement but there are definite signs of an uprising and potential overthrow by coup from my lower biceps and a couple of fingers that work in dysfunctional defiance. I believe absolutely that I'm improving – unlike a larger-than-life character in the centre who knows the future will only get worse.

Bola is a big black man from Nigeria with an even bigger laugh. He has problems with advanced arthritis in his hips, a mild stroke and an operation which has gone wrong. He isn't a well man. To get around he needs a stick and someone in attendance in case he has one of his dizzy spells.

Even though life is not going to get better he manages to invest happiness into every waking moment of his day, spreading warmth and candour evenly across all those he meets. Sure he's lazy, sure he's a little fruity with the ladies, sure he's terribly forgetful, yet the cumulative effect of the weeks I know him will live on. His cackle will always sit just behind my shoulder, booming out in raucous fashion like Long John Silver's parrot – a constant reminder that laughter is an essential component of the healing process.

We share an equal passion for *The Sopranos*. A good friend has supplied a boxed set of the first series of *The Sopranos* together with a DVD player on which we watch episode after episode back-to-back. If you don't know the programme then I commend it to you. It revolves around a New York Mafia mob headed up by one Tony Soprano who cries wolf with his psychoanalyst about the difficulties with his career which he euphemistically entitles 'construction'.

By night he goes out shooting people and by day he sits on a psychiatrist's couch ruminating on the teenage trials and tribulations of his 13-year-old son. The fretful father's concern – "I think he might be hanging out with the wrong kind of guys" – contrasts marvellously with the epic line uttered as he's about to push a rival hoodlum off a suspension bridge. "Consider yourself lucky, punk, I am in a good mood, I ain't going to shoot you on the way down."

I know all about the way down as, just to break the monotony, I fall over from time to time. This always coincides with the point in the day when I've either over-exerted myself in physiotherapy, or tried to move myself – or something – in haste. What I want to learn about now isn't the way down. It's the way home. There's nothing cruel intended in my heart but it's evident I've been hanging out with the wrong kind of guys.

8

Re-enter Stage Left

A Solitary Confinement

CHAPTER TWENTY-SEVEN

Re-enter Stage Left

I love the sound of autumn

Translucent noise in September.

Linament smells for sportsmen's thighs.

Turf that springs under foot and hoof.

Dewy and ripe, not sodden.

Breath condensed.

The first morning snuffle in the nose

Leaves that crackle, bursting with auburn burnish

Oxford indigo night sky

Splashed with ploughs and bears so bright

Glow-worms, unwitting, perform Swan Lake

Tortoise shells anoint faded lavenders

Bucolic hazes fade and imperatives appear

In the crushed concertina that is Libra and Scorpio

Things to be done, resolution, fitness beckons.

The year is starting - work can flow now -

Before crumpets and wood smoke enmesh our aspirations

In the charcoal, fug and brine of winter...

Anon

I am becoming distinctly unimpressed with hard floor surfaces as I keep landing on them. I'm desperate to swap polished lino floors for a bit of tufted Brinton. The vision of carpets overwhelms me one unsuspecting Tuesday as Suzi – now back to rude health – and I quietly slip away from the Wolfson, out of hospitals, out of rehabilitation and out of institutionalisation for what I hope will be forever.

Fat chance.

After ten months of hospital life I'm absolutely ready to come home. But while the boot camp regime is finally over I'm far from ready to be repatriated fully into society. There's a whole new status quo and a completely fresh set of partners, co-workers, supporters and carers to adjust to. As we drive home, (terraced house in the wilds of Fulham), carrying a significant volume of devices, props and equipment, the principal object I hope to render unnecessary at the earliest opportunity is the wheelchair.

Twenty years previously I'd been to Marrakesh. After dark coffees at the King's very own hotel, where staff walk along sweeping the gravel paths behind you, we turned out into the madness and mayhem of Jemaa el-Fna. The noise and smell hit us immediately, a multi-sensory assault including the sight of snake charmers, sultana pyramids, aromatic spices and mountains of delicious dates covered with flies. Stalls made out of crates had rough hewn sheets stretched above to protect traders from the harsh sun: a cauldron of excitement in this most vestigial primitive market square vibrating with colour, life and intrigue.

A broad-shouldered man 'walked' diagonally across the square on his knuckles. He'd lost both legs from the thigh downwards and strapped two old tractor tyres around the remaining stumps with pieces of string, enabling him to manoeuvre across the dusty surface like a giant gorilla. His gnarled knuckles were heavily calloused as they took the brunt of his weight. No one batted an eyelid. They were quite used to the vision of this quadruped moving with lithe power in his very own urban jungle. To him a wheelchair would have been a Rolls-Royce option, something he couldn't even imagine in a country too poor to consider the provision of a wheelchair as a basic standard of living. How dare we take such things for granted in our civilised culture? In a fit of absurd naivety,

I now want to be able to discard mine and dispatch it to a developing country where it will be treasured as a rare commodity.

Setting my target firmly to become independent as soon as possible, I want to walk whenever I can. It's crucial to graduate beyond the boundaries of stamina and balance which have, hitherto, prevented me from travelling very far on foot before resorting to the wheelchair for any journey of substance.

Each day I go to the park by the River Thames striving to increase the range and pace of my walking. Still using a Zimmer frame, my walking is hesitant over uneven surfaces on which falling leaves, twigs and yapping dogs become new opponents. I keep pushing my limits until one grey day when I'm too keen to complete the one-kilometre circuit around the park. My knees give out ten yards from my imaginary finishing line, the frame falls away from me and I sink on to my knees in exhaustion and self-pity. Suzi quickly finds volunteers. Two strangers help haul me up again and I shuffle my way to the car.

My frustration can be no more than short-lived as there's just too much assistance to call upon. If you know where and what to ask, an extraordinarily deep level of support is on offer. The local council is not going to let me back into society without help for the mind, body, sole and soul. The checklist goes on and on from such basic necessities as a bath board to a frame to sit around the loo with arm supports enabling me to get up from what's still a very low height. Can you imagine sitting on the loo and not being able to get up without someone to help you? Yes, I'm still that needy and utterly dependent on the clemency and compassion of friends and family.

Additional banisters are mounted on the staircase, commodes delivered and finger splints supplied, alongside specially adapted crutches with wide handles, and adjustable height trolleys so meals can be placed close enough to my chin to get the food in without dropping too much on the floor. And so the list goes on. A phalanx of physiotherapists, occupational therapists and social workers, as well as care workers and busybodies, queue at my door to book time in my weekly schedule, all helping me take the first tenuous steps of repatriation into the bigger world.

Kenneth, a Portuguese carer of African extraction, is assigned to visit me three times a day. For him I'm a bit of a treat. He has never come across a patient coming back from illness before. He specialises in tending terminals: those going the other way without hope of rediscovery or finding the person they used to be. Kenneth quickly becomes my friend. I grow to care about him as much as I grow to care about the fellow 'disenfranchisees' left in life's ashtray or wastepaper basket by savage illness and blight, who are swept up and plonked into the 'system'.

The HQ for their repatriation into an alternative life is Sunberry Day Care Centre near Fulham Football Club – a day-care facility for people with a wide variety of disabilities which provides an essential crutch to the middle section of their daily routine. Discarded by society because of their illness or infirmity, the building and its programmes help put a little self-respect and purpose back into their shaky world.

The centre's first wheel-bound patient to introduce himself is Philippe who does up his shirt's top button like a man of 75, draws multicoloured pictures with felt tip pens like a child of five and speaks to me in a covetous way as though we're both errant schoolboys of 15 who've just raided the tuck shop. He is, in fact, 45. At 25 he'd been in a motorcycle crash, leaving him with severe memory loss and paralysed from the waist down. When asking my name he explains he'll probably have to ask me again in another 'one five' minutes because no matter how many times I repeat the answer he'll not be able to remember it. This, from someone who speaks Italian, Spanish, German and French, underlines the tragedy and obscenity of his enforced sequestration.

He does, however, have one very interesting maxim which he applies when making any acquaintance. He studies whoever he's about to talk to and then tells that person about the things he has spotted which he most admires about their demeanour and dress. This should be a lovely way to guarantee he can provide some happiness and warmth to those looking after him. Most of the time it works well, but one of the other faculties Philippe lost in the accident is how to differentiate between rude and polite. Thus "Good morning Margaret, I admire your cashmere cardigan and compassionate countenance" starts off well enough before taking a horrendous wrong turn with "Your sultry smile, sweet smell and lovely big bouncy tits." I like Philippe.

The community bus picks me up most mornings and zig-zags its way to the centre in Fulham where the waifs and strays, malcontents and unfortunates have the quality of their lives marginally improved by a medley of activities. They while away their days nourished by the care, love and attention of an army of philanthropically minded social workers. The building appears to have been designed to induce gloom but, despite its best attempts, isn't allowed to succeed – the ethos and spirit of the team working there won't allow it. I'm deposited here to wait for the next bus on the relay to collect me and several other hardy souls who want to conquer the equipment at the Douglas Bader Centre gymnasium across the Thames in Roehampton – a special-purpose facility for the disabled and those who have lost limbs. Conversation's always a bit hit and miss because you're never quite sure whether the person you're talking to can remember who you are. And in some cases who they are.

Once on the bus a different culture wraps itself around you. It's the sort of bus that as children we used to chuck v-signs at while the 'spasos' went past. Now I'm on the inside poking my tongue out and waiting for any sign of digital insurrection. My fellow passengers form a patchwork of deprivations. There's William, ten years into his Parkinson's disease, whose every move seems so tortured. His gait suggests he is a special adviser to the Ministry of Silly Walks, so over-exaggerated has his stride become to compensate for the debilitation of his illness. Sometimes his perpetual twisting and turning stops as he goes into 'the refrigerator' – the frozen pose endured by people with the condition. This can last two minutes or two hours, you can't hurry it or break it. You just have to wait. To me it looks rather frightening but to William it's just another inconvenience to tag on to the bottom of his long list. When his body is ready, and not before, it releases its grip and his heavily compromised participation in life starts again.

William likes cigarettes and sick jokes. The sicker the better. His favourite involves an old man admitted to a nursing home who is befriended by a lady called Doris. Each afternoon she makes him a cup of tea before placing her hand under his nightshirt and holding his willy, while he sits on the edge of his bed. Doris is distraught when she realises she has been usurped by another patient, Mabel. She confronts her former beau by asking him what Mabel has got that she hasn't. "She makes me a cup of tea like you used to," he replies, "and she puts her hand under my nightshirt to hold my willy just like you used to. But now it's much more exciting because she has Parkinson's." Coming from anybody else this joke would be deemed to be in very bad taste. Coming from William you have to laugh – crying would hurt too damn much.

There's Dan the Dustman who can't read or write but compensates fully for his lack of such skills by talking the hind legs off as many donkeys as he can find. He craves attention and affection, and wants to put smiles on people's faces – it's his way of coping – yet he consistently misses the mark. At 62 he has, by his own account, a highly desirable collection of toy cars and trains but insufficient boxes to put them in. My donation of empty Ferrero-Rocher clear plastic boxes, to display the toys, reduces him to tears. Dan does not live in a world overly blessed with kindness. Please don't ask who gave me the full boxes in the first place; they have their pride.

We all have our own methods to get by. Some are constantly introspective, others absurdly loquacious. It's every man for himself in the 'how to survive disability battle zone'. No matter how much lifestyle coaching you offer anyone, there's no one easy way to compensate for levels of debility that turn your world upside down. Take young Keely. Aged 20 she'd fallen off a roof and broken her back, to then learn she was paralysed from her stone-encrusted tummy button down and would never walk again. You can tell she's yielding to it; the stomach for a fight isn't there. Oblivious to the impact her lack of endeavour in exercise is having on her body – and her constitution – she tries to get by, pretending nothing life-changing has happened.

Until she announces she's pregnant, that is, and the father has done a runner. This is a shock and awkward surprise to all who know her. Who in all conscience would want to get a woman, already in such a medically parlous state, 'with child'? And how in any God's name do they think she'll be able to give a baby a future worth having? It beggars all belief.

Inside the Douglas Bader Centre's gymnasium I often encounter a number of other sorry tales. All tug at the heart strings in equal measure. Mandy, now 60, was diagnosed with MS at 23. She has four children, all of whom take great pride in looking after her and making what's left of her life as tolerable as possible. Every day she goes to the gym to fight her illness and keep it as far at bay as possibe. It's a titanic battle. The MS is resolutely trying to retain its stranglehold on her disposition every bit as much as she's determined to prevent it from taking her life over completely.

Her walking style mimics a tepee. Using two sticks she spreads her legs out straight at 45 degrees behind and apart, while plonking the sticks at a similar jaunt ahead. Going for a stroll is a thing of her distant past, getting across a room now a military campaign. You can see the torture etched across her face as she sits upon the rowing machine – her hands wrapped in Velcro so she can grip the handles – and pulls the weights, a movement that enables her shoulders to flex and stretch. She's a real fighter, someone who never moans about her lot: a stunning example of strength in adversity.

You'd hope your family doctor could help you find this greater strength. But I've never felt so utterly detached from my GP as I do in today's society. Indeed I'm determined that if I ever have any signs of anything mildly serious ever again, I'll go straight to my nearest Accident and Emergency department. If the police forces move their stations there too, who knows what else will follow? Perhaps I'll buy my petrol, have my fingerprints checked, leave a blood sample and collect my weekly groceries at the same time.

Certainly we need to overhaul the outdated and perfunctory collection of Britain's hospital buildings. Yet did we intend, in all conscience, to imbalance the relationship between preventative medicine and care – last provided by community doctors a generation ago – by so openly encouraging people to go straight to hospital? My own experience teaches me that unless I want a placebo or to waste time with my GP, who'll only refer me to a specialist anyway, I might just as well admit myself directly. Your average GP's bright and armed with years of training and knowledge. He or she, like most thoroughbred creatures, needs exercise, particularly for the brain.

- CHAPTER TWENTY-EIGHT -
Re-enter Stage Left

Friends and relations continue to visit, some from as far away as America and Hong Kong. They still have to negotiate around my physiotherapy sessions which take up about 20 hours a week, but it's so much nicer to welcome people into your own environment and to allow their health of body and mind to encourage, infect and nurture you.

One gives me a DVD, *The Motorcycle Diaries* – the story of an idealistic, educated, charismatic and handsome young man who postpones his medical training to take a journey of discovery around South America. After volunteering in a leper colony, he never returns home, banishing any craven thoughts and joining the guerrillas in Cuba. He was Che Guevara: the revolutionary who swapped the roistering good time sampled while travelling in the Andes for a life of attrition that was prematurely terminated.

There's plenty of piety and poetry in the film but its raw beauty lies in the exploration of the continent with his best friend and their battle with nature, lack of money and the vagaries of a 1939 Norton 500's engine. It's truly thought-provoking – is leprosy worse than one's own condition? – and should be essential viewing for anyone who has suffered an illness.

Of course, it's also a wonderfully photogenic escape for an armchair traveller. While I've no yen to join any Central American rebels, it's the type of gloriously free-wheeling journey I can't contemplate at the moment. Indeed, I still can't tie my own shoelaces properly, or undo the buttons on my shirt. I can, however, lift my arms in the air and give an approximate impression of a normal person shaking hands. The only difference appears to be 'Are you in the Masons?', a question I'm invariably asked when disengaging hands, as my index finger curls in on itself, getting squashed in the shake. It's compounded by an inability to retrieve my hand, as my thumb wraps itself around the back of the hand of any poor innocent soul joining me for the handshake dance.

To correct this and my other malfunctions I flex my finger and hand muscles, waking them from their torpor whenever I can. It's a great way to pass the time on journeys, including our jaunts on the sensory bus, so called because it beeps when reversing towards cars, walls and other objects. I admit I'd hoped for something more winsome when first espying the word *sensory* on the side of vehicle. A melange of aromatherapy oils, music by Enya and some scented candles with rose petal water might make our journey along the South Circular Road a softer, more serene experience.

We touch our forelocks to the daily sight of a shrine to the much lamented, died too young, driving his Mini too fast, lived life to the full under the influence of hallucinogenics whilst riding a white swan, Marc Bolan. Pictures of him in his King Charles I wig, in full makeup with star dust sprinkled in his heavily-tressed locks, still adorn two trees near Barnes railway station. It's a display of such glittering tackiness that even a magpie would be ashamed.

It induces silent contemplation. Is it better to die young? How much less idealised would our opinions be of Marc Bolan or Princess Diana if they'd turned 50, suffered a stroke and lost the use of one side of their body along with the ability and will to speak? These thoughts ride with me on the way back to the Douglas Bader Gym. The facility is far busier since the devastating London bombings of 7th July. The resultant carnage made global headlines but the real impact can be measured in the faces and empty stares of the victims trying to rebuild their shattered lives at this very gymnasium. To have your legs blown off, lose an eye and your best friend and still retain your love of all mankind is a big ask.

Yet no sooner have I entered the building than a young woman in her early thirties – with two new metal legs attached from the thigh downwards – strides past me using crutches. She's giggling. Her shorts expose the pipework, ducting and intricacies of the new metal limbs. Complete with trainers wrapped around her false feet she might be excused a moment of self-pity. Yet here she is, in a state of high excitement, roaring with laughter as a lugubrious technician follows behind her holding a can of oil and a large screwdriver. "I think your right leg is moving a bit slow," he exclaims. "Sit down for goodness sake!" She has no reason to bless 7th July and every excuse to curse it, but she's damned if she's going to stop enjoying her life.

The uplifting scene contrasts wildly with my forays back into mainstream life. I'm trying to split my week from a disabled one on Mondays, Wednesdays and Fridays to an able-bodied one on Tuesdays and Thursdays. So it's the first Tuesday of the month when we venture out to eat as preparation for the much larger and more real challenge of returning to work.

My favourite restaurant in England is Bibendum, housed on the first floor of the old Michelin building in west London. Although lovely at night I prefer it at lunchtime when sunshine streams in through its stained glass windows spreading dappled light across the high ceiling. Violets, indigos, petrol blues, emerald apples and chiffon yellows dance on your tablecloth and glassware. Its tables are never set too close together, its food is always sharp, simple, well observed and bloody good. The service can be a bit French at times – you know, stuffy, supercilious and a bit up itself – but on the whole I just like the space.

This outing is a late low-key celebration of a birthday as I'd not been strong enough to venture out on the day itself which arrived soon after leaving the Wolfson. Two great friends join us and the occasion goes swimmingly; that is until the point at the end of the meal when I need to go to the loo. We've made the mistake of selecting a pair of proper trousers with a zip on the front, belt and buckle. Rank bad planning on my part, I confess. There isn't a disabled toilet on the same floor and Suzi feels uncomfortable taking me into the gents.

We excuse ourselves to the ladies present in their loo on our way in, as though it's a perfectly normal routine for a disabled man on sticks like some postprandial ritual. Getting into the narrow cubicle is difficult enough, but the harder part is doing my trousers up when I've finished. I can't do it myself so I hiss instructions while Suzi squats down to get my fly at her eye level. You might be thinking this is starting to look a bit saucy. Perhaps there are parallels with Boris Becker turning a broom cupboard at the Metropolitan Hotel into the most frequently requested space in the building – and also, given his subsequent divorce, the most expensive British letting space ever in cost per square inch.

I'm desperately trying to think about anything else than inches that might be squaring up when the cubicle is barged open. "Disgusting!" exclaims the intemperate harridan. "On what possible basis can you justify such salacious behaviour? Get out now before I report you to the authorities!"

I confess the evidence doesn't look too good. As the officer of the toilet police vents her spleen, Suzi's hand is stuck inside my zip, her mouth wide open in horror and she's licking her lips – she always sticks out her tongue when concentrating (honestly!). To compound the fellony I'm smiling with sapient pleasure after an epicurean feast in the dining room. A deep breath and we rise above the kerfuffle, leaving the ladies' loo with our heads held high and a suitably pithy riposte to the verbal assault. "Thank you so much for introducing yourself, the pleasure is all ours." I now plan my choice of the right trousers as studiously as the route of any gourmet tour.

On a later able-bodied Thursday I head out for a rather different dining experience. I'm going to a friend's house for al fresco supper by the river. I first met Martin on a boys' golfing trip to the Caribbean when we played a round on the first day and he forgot the sun cream. He tried to see the funny side when the guys all ordered lobster for breakfast the following day, before – wearing a long-sleeved shirt, two gloves and a wide-brimmed hat – he gamely tried to play again as his arms, nose and neck turned an even brighter pink. We've kept in touch regularly over the years and now Martin announces he's going to collect me and take me to his house for dinner.

The chauffeur arrives in an anthracite grey Bentley Mulsanne Turbo. It is, without doubt, a great car. It's great because the boot takes a Zimmer frame and a wheelchair at the same time, while its doors are so wide you can swing your legs in and, better still, adjust the seat height. Next time you see one go past and think to yourself 'flash bastard' – or even worse 'footballer' – just remember that if my fantasy society ever becomes reality, they'll be standard issue to the disabled, while able-bodied folk will have to cram themselves into a Mini or 2CV.

The meal by the river is a triumph of ambition over logic. I can't get down the pathway without being carried, lifted or pushed. At least my trousers hold firm. Martin meanwhile, as well as being a Shintu priest, travel agent and bundle of frenetic energy, is turning his attentions to Albania and its forgotten vineyards. A much more interesting topic than Polish plumbers for our cappuccino classes to debate, don't you think? What about kicking off your next pretentious dinner party by asking, "How is your erectile function?" closely followed by, "I was talking to my Albanian viniculturist the other day."

If laughing at myself, laced with rants against disabled body prejudices, is a key ingredient in the mental recovery recipe, then relentless physiotherapy is my guiding bible for physical improvement. Mondays have become the local workout morning. I go to a different gym half a mile from the house and place my welfare in the hands of Paul, a cheerful über-fit east Londoner who, for the last decade, has specialised in guiding disabled folks like me. A freelancer, he cycles from gym to gym, and must help over 200 people each week, darting from one venue to the next. Yet he also knows how to make me feel I'm the most important man in the world. He's absolutely the sort of bloke who should receive an MBE for unsung hero activities.

CHAPTER TWENTY-NINE

Re-enter Stage Left

I f Monday mornings are for the body, Monday afternoons are for work. Yes, after 11 months it's now time to get the brain back into gear and see if I can be of any value to the directors I'd so inconsiderately dropped in it all those eons ago. A couple of hours a week may seem laughable but it's a start and it allows me a peek at the problems women experience when they depart their work desk to have babies, leaving all their confidence behind in the in-tray. Before this moment I have, in my male blinkered stupidity, assumed work is like riding a horse. Fall off and you get straight back on. That's poppycock. You also leave your knowledge, contacts, pace, brio and relevance behind.

Assuming a role of importance again will require patience and indulgence from my work colleagues, along with their permission, of course. But picking up the threads of what's relevant is much scarier. How dare I? How can I possibly offer pertinent advice, let alone instruction, when I've been in another universe for so long? And that's the crux of my 'how to get on with workmates' dilemma. How to master the client challenge will take new bravery pills and lots of trial and error.

Physically my present status quo simply isn't enough. Increasingly impatient with the daily exercises to stimulate nerve endings, I'm ready to try something more exotic. Rations of working life for starters and alternative medical devices for main course. I meet up with Dr Roberto Ciaff, which is not Italian for Chav. For 25 years he has been combining his qualifications in medicine with a fascination for electronic engineering. Initially targeting motor neurone patients he has perfected a method of sending electric impulses through the body to enhance the pace of regeneration in the nervous system.

Our early exchanges don't fill me with supreme confidence. I'm invited to put my feet into a bucket of water and am linked up to the national grid to receive a variety of electric impulses, a process then repeated on my hands. Miraculously the pain in my fingers abates. Not forever, but just enough to remind me what it feels like to enjoy something approaching normal sensation.

I switch from doubting Thomas to disciple in an instant. It's the first of countless weekly pilgrimages to Oxted. We progress from bucket immersion to direct application of pads to the spine, thighs and elbows, with a variety of positive and negative pulses coursing through my veins. The different components of my electronic workout are even given code names: Plus and Minus, Left and Right Boogie, Marching up the Hill and The Tumble Dryer. The machinery lets me take my legs on a far longer route march than if I try to walk, and while there's no cardiovascular benefit it's surprising to feel the effect that an electric impulse targeted, say, on the knee has on the shoulder.

The principles of acupuncture still apply but the best analogy to describe the effect of Dr Ciaff's technology is a foot pressed firmly down on a hosepipe with the tap turned on full blast. It accumulates pressure – exactly how the hibernating parts of my body feel before the treatment. The electrical impulses then drill away at blockages until key nerves wake up, releasing the reservoir of energy which has built up behind the dam. In essence the foot has been lifted off the hosepipe.

At the beginning most settings are at maximum to get as much juice through my system as possible to clear the debris. As time progresses I can only tolerate relatively small doses because areas of sensitivity are being rediscovered. Target areas enlarge because the motorways carrying messages from brain to target and back again have been cleared by the technology's highway patrol.

By happenstance I miss a few weeks and realise how addicted I've become to the process and resultant buzz. The system works by providing temporary relief at the very least and might, I suspect, become standard procedure for treatment of people with wasting illnesses like MS as the wider medical profession accepts the process. It's already second nature to sports teams whose thoroughbred athletic torsos require the finest of fine-tuning. It's not just steroids and muscle bulking agents for our professional sportsmen these days.

The electric workout is here to stay. But what I want to know is, am I here to stay or is some sort of ending in sight? Christmas is fast approaching. Anniversary time. A time to give enormous thanks I'm still here, much improved by comparison to this time last year. I have most of my Christmas cards ready to post, presents allocated and wrapped, and as the shortest day of the year, 21st December, breaks I proffer a little prayer to all my gods for their forbearance.

For 12 months now I have been sidelined to the emergency pit stop whilst the rest of the world races by. Can you please stop the world? I want to get back on. It's not possible yet, I'm afraid. I can only manage to undo shoelaces but can't do them up. I can put food into my mouth with a spoon but can't cut it with a knife. I can undo some buttons on my shirt but can't get my left arm into the sleeve or do up any buttons. The list goes on, something and nothing, so near and so far.

Parts of my body almost look normal. My hands and feet receive messages intermittently, offering pain and imprecision as their excuse for not writing home. My trunk, back and sides, I assume, are reasonably OK because they don't hurt as much, yet even they're not tuned into the precise frequency. Fertile bits, growing back to their previous reality, are matched by patches of wasteland that remain barren in terms of response.

A year is a long time. Quite long enough to document before I lose your attention. My patience is wearing thinner. As I approach being able to do something correctly, so my temper shortens. The time when I had no choice but to abdicate sovereignty over my frame is long past. Tantalisingly, my faculties are returning in random order and it's supremely frustrating trying to allot independence to functions like walking and writing when neither is yet roadworthy to pass their MOT.

Meanwhile and elsewhere, Sundance is at home in sheltered accommodation, confined to bed on some days, able to walk freely on others, but inspired by his children as ever. He's looking for romance in Whitby where he has met a fellow MS sufferer who's rather sweet on him. They're busy perfecting what he calls 'The Lovemaker's Guide to Romance in Wheelchairs' which is sure to be a bestseller. Before you ask, yes, it's best to use at least two chairs in the process.

The crew at the hospital in Bath are much the same except for the introduction of a new matron who is busy dishing out the orders, same as the old matron. Plus ça change. Kirsten is now a stalker. Having followed her boyfriend's change of jobs she has moved to London to take over the local outpatient supervision programme and – to our joint surprise – is awarded me as her first case. She is the most welcome sight. Tears of unbounded pleasure cascade down my snivelling face.

Her arrival brings vivid memories flooding back. Particularly the recollection of a trip – suggested by Kirsten – which Suzi and I made to celebrate the first six months of my recovery: an excellent afternoon adventure in a 'taxi'. It was actually a small minibus with an electric ramp enabling wheelchairs to be pushed up and inside in one movement, providing my first chance to explore the world beyond the hospital campus.

We'd been invited out to tea by a handsome woman called Lisa. Thirty-two years previously, as the owner of a restaurant near Bath, she had the great misfortune to employ me as an ancillary waiter. I hadn't seen her for years but, to my surprise, I spied her turning into the corridor on her way to visit another patient. It was her idea we should visit her stunning 16th century house in a hidden valley just outside Bath – a perfect blend of solitude and proximity. Wheelchair access was hopeless so her partner Donald heaved me in through the front door. The quintessential English summer's day demonstrated perfectly why we always discuss the weather. The sun emerged sporadically amidst dark clouds, interrupted by a magnificent gleaming rainbow, while the logs on the fire crackled, spat and smoked, and we sipped Earl Grey tea – mine through a straw – and savoured the freshest cucumber sandwiches.

Interestingly, the man who Lisa had been visiting in hospital was her immediate neighbour in the valley. Christopher, in his early sixties, had been struck down by a stroke. It was awful timing: one daughter was due to give birth to his first grandchild, the other about to get married. So determined was he to walk one daughter down the aisle and attend the birth with the other that Christopher overdosed on physiotherapy.

Never mind his neuralgia, or the moments when he fell over, he was serious competition. Until then I'd thought I was the one showing the most cussed determination. Valentine, his redoubtable and charming wife, had no idea what an inspiration her husband was, making me double my efforts. She also lent me cassette tapes ranging from a bit of Le Carré to Samuel Pepys' diaries, doubling the rations of food for the brain.

Rations of love are an entirely different matter, however. I've been so poor at handing any out. I remember how long it took my younger son to come to terms with the fact I was so unwell. It was at the six-month turning point when, on the point of leaving my bedside one sultry afternoon, he asked me how I cleaned my teeth. "Someone does it for me," I replied. He nodded and then asked, "And how do you put your clothes on?" I repeated "Someone does it for me."

It was as though a penny was finally dropping. All the love he'd offered unconditionally had been based on a suspension of reality. Dad is supposed to be there to rely upon, to be solid and dependable – and I wasn't doing a very good job of convincing him of my strength or durability. A six-month sojourn had turned into 12, missing out on him entering his 18th year, wrestling with his A-levels and choosing further education: time I can never get back or reverse.

His original artwork, for which he claimed the school's golden paintbrush award no less, is the cover of this book. It's his way of showing support. He finds it easier to talk to his art master about my health than he does to my face – a sentiment I totally understand.

Not to be outdone by Charlie, my elder son Sam bashes out a few records to an innocent My Space public including a track called 'Heart'. He's full of it. And in her own way their mother, and my first wife George, is as supportive and helpful as I have any right to expect, let alone hope for. She has performed so many acts of mercy and assistance behind the scenes that if I thank her for each one it will take me till tomorrow.

Yet I know tomorrow can only belong to me – and I can only lead a truly healthy life – if I adopt a fresh mindset and learn from the experience of others. One piece of advice stands out. It came from an articulate and vital young man who'd broken his back diving into a shallow swimming pool, spending eight months cocooned inside a plaster cast that prevented the slightest movement. Yet this state of abject surrender didn't stop him from making a full recovery and returning to his former high-octane existence.

So when he speaks, I listen. Intently. He's one of my few visitors with experience of long-term debilitation. His speech is considered and precise as he debunks the assumptions I've made about recovery. "When you're better and someone asks 'How are you?', just say 'Fine thank you,'" he tells me. "You'll want to explain every last detail and won't see how quickly their eyes glaze over. You'll not be box office news for any length of time, believe me. People just won't want to know."

My quandary now is to determine at what time to announce to the world I'm on the way back. So I set an arbitrary point – exactly one year after my admission to the first hospital – reasoning that by announcing I'm better, a level of self-fulfilment will kick in the more I repeat the phrase.

Granted I still need a lot of help from Kenneth the kindly care worker. He wakes me each morning and enables me to take increasing responsibility for my own ablutions. Agreed, I can't use my hands properly to dial a telephone number or write an almanac of the last year. You are right to observe I still can't dress myself, handle loose change or make a hot drink on my own. The authorities won't allow me to drive and my paperwork confirms I'm disabled. But even though my body is ameliorating at a slower pace than my mindset – and there are years of relentless physiotherapy still to come – I'm not prepared to wait any longer.

This story needs a happy ending and society will just have to ignore the lack of sartorial elegance, my gait which resembles The Tin Man from *The Wizard of Oz* and my sporadic lack of zest. I'm learning to play bridge and although I can't deal, shuffle, or even hold my cards, it doesn't stop me playing. When I first arrive at the card school I can see the other novices staring at me in trepidation as I inch towards them on my walking frame. As they cup their hands across their mouths, I suspect they're whispering to their immediate neighbour, "Please don't let the freak sit next to me."

There was a time when this would have made me timorous. Not any more. This is the point where I want to stop being classed as 'off sick'. It may only be a psychological sleight of hand, or mind, but it's enough. I'm recovered sufficiently to consign my 50th year to its own resting place. From hereon in I want to be treated as a well person. So please don't ask me any more questions. The only answer you will get is "Just fine, thank you."

9

Ashes to Anger

A Solitary Confinement

CHAPTER THIRTY

Ashes to Anger

O r it would have been "just fine thank you". But then my dad dies. He's a big man, 6'8" in his prime, yet a gentle gentleman in all his manners. He literally runs out of breath at the end, having been in and out of hospital for most of the year since turning 90. Last Thursday he rallied but on the Friday his breathing dipped alarmingly and he was ambulanced to the A&E department of the Bristol Royal Infirmary. They're keeping him alive until we, his family, can get there but the sepsis is so overwhelming he can no longer breathe unsupported.

So, surrounded by his loved ones, we hold his hand, tell him we'll always be with him and watch him literally run out of puff and slip away. He's become terribly hot so a fan has been placed close to him, making his white hair stick out and waft upwards in the breeze. It keeps moving after he's left us, still trying to make us smile with his unwitting Mr Pastry impersonation. I'm sure he continues to laugh and smile upon us even now.

His 50 years of unconditional love gave me my moral compass, which I fight to observe, along with a fund of stories, jokes, asides and observations I'll never forget. He witnessed two world wars, the Suez Crisis and the Falklands War, along with the invasion of Iraq, and the birth of television and the Internet, while sticking blissfully to his golden era in which the omnipotent Bing Crosby ruled the airwaves. He was also a compassionate man. I've learned from his lesson. Put the anger back in its box. In short, he was the best dad and friend I could have hoped for.

And now he's gone. The utter futility and sense of loss should have been easy to predict and plan for, but I feel overwhelmed, destitute, trapped and very, very angry. In short, I'm anything but fine. Why the huge breadth of change in my mood? Let me try to explain.

Despite all my reslience and apparent recovery, my body no longer fits my frame. It's as if I've picked up someone else's coat when leaving a restaurant – and will do so every day for the rest of my life. While my sight, hearing and taste are relatively intact, my sense of smell is completely shot, with touch returning at snail's pace through miniscule shards of improvement. My heart is older – my behaviour occasionally fast forwards to that of a septuagenarian – while arousal is off the agenda, my body more an erroneous than erogenous zone. It makes me furious. But I've made the decision to move forward. Like all the barriers surmounted previously, they're there to be scaled, broken, removed or torn down.

All this changes with Dad's death. Calm acceptance of my lot goes down the proverbial toilet. The emotional tsunami is from a different ocean but, like the Atlantic storm that hit me last December, it turns nasty. Very nasty. The world I've tried so hard to rebuild comes crashing down all over again. The futility of all my efforts to put life back on to an even keel are laid bare for open inspection.

A big black hole engulfs me and I dive down into the very depths of myopic despondence. Why now? Couldn't you just have let me be a bit stronger to get back to caring for him? How can I be expected to write an obituary, organise a funeral, invite all his friends and relations, book the wake and do those bastard shoelaces up?

I don't want to be trapped here in an alien body when I so desperately need all my faculties back. The solitary confinement is under renewed assault. Yes, my body most certainly has been attacked but my mind has not given in, until now. I'm so bleedingly, contemptuously, splenetically and profoundly angry because, buried as they had been, Dad's death finally makes the suppressed boils of emotional bile and contempt erupt, exploding like the most brutal volcano.

For all my self-pity and protestations it has been a calm mind with which I've learned to reconnect with all the love I mistakenly thought had disappeared into cold storage all those months ago. It has taken time and great patience but the love of life and giving to others has filtered through. Drawn perhaps by osmosis or morphed by Mr Spock, it has come back in wave after wave. And now this.

It's shaken me to the core. The loss of any unconditional love is always a shock because to receive it in the first place is such a bonus and certainly not our birthright. The sadness of his passing makes me feel worse for sure. Down and down goes the mood, blacker and blacker turns the sky.

Yet, perhaps inevitably, just as the storm clouds break, so a freshness emerges. The rage begins slowly to subside. A certainty he'll always be at my side gradually washes over me in tandem with, but outweighing, the waves of melancholy. Before I realise it, I make a subconscious decision. I'll finally stop writing this book and feeling so selfishly sorry for myself. I'll look forward with new purpose. It was, and still is, my father's giving of strength to others which takes the lid off my coffin.

Even though the responsibility curve had swung its full arc years before and I've been his carer for ages, this most recent passage had made us brothers in infirm arms. It was an equalisation: confirmation that I could now mimic his mannerisms with impunity. They'd been genetically absorbed, but I'd fought so hard to subconsciously deny the inheritance. At last this self-deception is no longer necessary. The trap is broken.

On the Monday after his death in Bristol I head back to south London for an operation. It means returning to the hospital where they sewed my head together after a fall. I'm not looking forward to it, but nothing prepares me for the sight of three policemen in flak jackets brandishing semi-automatic weapons next to the room where I'm waiting for surgeons to correct another impediment.

This very morning there has been a 'Shootin' in Tootin' outside the hospital. They fear reprisals. It doesn't help my sense of inner calm or sphincter control – the part of me about to be reduced from its greedy dual status. Any hint of anger here will be quoshed instantly so I cheer myself up by attributing a new line to my ridiculous hero, Ricky Tomlinson: 'security, my arse!'

I need a day to recover from the anaesthetic, tentatively perching on comfy cushions before we can get down to the very serious business of organising a fitting tribute. We hold the funeral service a few days later and thoughts of crying are absented. The day's a triumph of organisation and cooperation from all our friends and helpers. It passes into history as it does for all families, and the tears of sadness, joy and relief come, thankfully, when everyone has gone home.

Suzi does everything in her power to lift me out of the abyss. We have much to be grateful for. But it's still here: the prison without bars, the sense of a solitary confinement. Other illnesses may come and go but few pervade like GBS with its limpet-like desire to stick around. It has made me invisible to many, some stare straight through me, others ignore me: a reflection of my self-regard perhaps, but an ignominy unplanned for sure. It has imposed huge restrictions on others, permanently diverting the course of their lives. Along with removing my sense of smell and touch, it has triggered problems with my walking and removed my independence while devastating my sex drive and energy levels, and introducing years of relentless physiotherapy. It has made me totally reconsider how to explain myself in business, supplied untold pain as my one abiding constant, and removed me from my children. My dress code is changed forever, as is the way I regard others' boorish behaviour. It has even separated my body and mind. It has been one hell of an epiphany.

But I am going to beat it, no matter how long it takes.

Lest you think me still sad though, let me leave you with a smile. Try to picture the changes needed in the frequency and nature of going on holiday now forced upon us. That I can even take a holiday makes me a lucky man, of course. I have got back into the work saddle, given myself permission to take charge and worked out how to behave in sufficiently normal a way in business that I can safely say "I'm back". On conditional discharge perhaps, but definitely back.

And that means holidays are too. When Suzi and I get on a plane we now use a wheelchair – it's too far for me to walk from public transport to the terminal. So I try not to let my pride get in the way of practicality. In fact the man assigned to get us on board is fast approaching and guess what? He only has one arm. But remember, it's the only one that works properly between us.

I contemplate saying something sympathetic but it doesn't come out that way. I recall how the children playing in the Wimbledon park would have reacted and, somehow, it just pops out: a sentence under new public ownership. "But I don't want to go around in circles."

At first there's silence. Then very very slowly, he begins to laugh. We laugh. The couple next to us start to laugh. The queue behind us laughs. And then the whole departure lounge appears to snigger aloud to this hopelessly incorrect jest.

It serves as an essential reminder. Yes, life can be cruel at times but – following the doctrine that there's always someone worse off than yourself – you must count your blessings. Give thanks for them, no matter how small. No one said life was easy, but determination, persistence, anger harnessed in the right way and, above all, patience will take you such a long way. After all, doesn't GBS stand for Getting Better Slowly?

The Ten-Year Itch

"The end of all our exploring will be to arrive where we
started and know the place for the first time."

T.S. Eliot

If Guillain-Barré is a journey, my outward leg began amidst the Victorian solidity of Isambard Brunel's Paddington station and carried me all the way to St Ives. The return, however, encountered signal and track problems outside Basingstoke. I'm still there, stranded amongst its myriad roundabouts.

Hello. Welcome back. A decade after promising I'd put my pen down for the last time, I've decided to send another – don't worry, most definitely final – dispatch from the front line. Before I bring you news of my fellow passengers, a little personal update.

As I say, my return journey, for the moment at least, has ended frustratingly short of its departure point. Even allowing for the fact that none of us escape the ravages of time, I can't claim to be the same person I was when this tale began all those years ago. Psychologically and emotionally there is no going back. It's not possible to undergo such a draining, exhausting, at times bewildering experience and re-emerge untouched.

How has my body bounced back? Well, regular and copious physio from Eddie, a warm, generous and talented therapist, has reaped rich rewards. I mastered driving again, providing enormous and hugely welcome independence. I can also dress myself although lack the fingertip strength to close my top button and knot a tie.

My balance is not fully restored. Once a week I fall over for no particular reason. Clearly, while communications between my feet, which 'slap' occasionally as I walk, and my brain are better than Trump's White House, they perhaps fall short of Tory Party HQ (although you do wonder sometimes). If you recall my metaphor of accidentally picking up someone else's coat when leaving a restaurant, it still applies to my body. I've never managed to track down and slip on my old garment. I'm still wearing someone else's and the damn thing doesn't quite fit.

So much for my health. What about my home? Suzi and I have swapped the tightly-packed, ever-inflating terraced streets of Fulham for the bucolic air and wide rolling valleys of the Cotswolds. It might not help my miscommunicating sole but it just has to be good for my soul. It was terribly difficult telling Eddie we were leaving to live the country life – it's one hell of a commute from Elephant and Castle, just south of the Thames, to north of Woodstock by 7am. We're still in regular contact but his restorative stretching and manipulation sessions are collateral damage from our move.

England's green and pleasant land isn't the only tonic, mind you. We've bought a flat in Majorca which we adore, and now worship the sun twice a year, breathing in herb-and honey-scented Mediterranean air and eating some superb Iberian food: a regular recharge for the system.

Events have moved even faster on the work front. So much has happened over the preceding decade, it's hard to know where to begin – and whether any of it is a lateral product of my fall, decline and rise from GBS. After disagreeing with other shareholders in our hotel management company, we bought them out and I am now chairman – the best career move I've ever made. I returned to full-time work and the company has expanded dramatically. Bespoke now embraces over 200 properties and is looking to distant warmer horizons, stretching its embrace to include India, Morocco, Dubai, where we have opened an office, and Singapore.

We've also had the chance to convert two striking historic buildings into fabulous 'storytelling' hotels. Not sure what that is? Well, allow yourself a five-minute break and google Hotel Gotham. You'll see how a Manchester Art Deco masterpiece designed by Edwin Lutyens, once full of bankers, has been reinvented as a slice of vintage 'Manc-hattan' complete with flamboyant cast of period characters. It has performed the unique double of simultaneously being crowned 'hottest' and 'coolest' UK hotel. I was the driving force behind the venture, so clearly, in the long term, GBS doesn't stifle one's creative flair!

It's exciting dynamic stuff but I've also had some rather wonderful reminders of my working life from well before this whole episode started. I was recently in North Wales near Llandudno and dropped into beautiful Bodysgallen Hall. You may remember it from when I was first lying in intensive care and 'flashed back' to a cushy life in luxury hotels, recalling my opening it in 1981. Well it's still there, still rather beautiful and, remarkably, the same lady is still running the restaurant. The circle of life may have turned a few more notches but somehow we managed to recognise each other after 35 years: a lovely moment.

So much for me, now how about some of the others who've graced the stage in this play of several acts? As you might expect, much life has happened around me over the last ten years. There has been a lot of it going on. An awful lot.

For starters there has been a marriage. My elder son, Sam, came to live with us after graduating from university with the aim of taking a master's degree at University College London. Then one day he announced he was leaving. Leaving his bedroom, leaving the house, leaving London. In fact he was heading to South Korea where he was going to teach English to young children.

Without a single sign of homesickness he extended his one-year contract into a second year and promptly fell in love. He married in the South Korean port of Busan and my daughter-in-law Injin has come to England to live in south London and find a variety of jobs. One day she came to our house with her mother and aunt for tea. Not just a cuppa but a full afternoon high tea replete with scones and cream, crumpets, blackcurrant jam and Madeira cake. At this point the story goes into s-l-o-w m-o-t-i-o-n. As we looked on in horror, auntie pulled her jam-covered knife out of the jar and, without breaking stride, smothered a deep slick of blackcurrant on top of her cucumber sandwich. Our flailing arms were too slow. Into her mouth went the groundbreaking culinary fusion and out came her judgment: "Dericious."

There have also been births, none of which are down to me but on Suzi's side, where there are now no less than five grandchildren. They mainly come with pretty far-out christian names, namely a Wolfe, a Rafferty and a Kit Fox, all on her son's side, while on her daughter's side there's now a Rocky. Thankfully little Olive appeared on the day of my 60th birthday rendering any mention of my future birthdays obsolete. No sign of children from Charlie, my youngest boy, but Sam and Injin have produced a baby boy called Maximilian, a heady combo of South Korean and Cheltenham, with a sweet smile!

And, as is the nature of life, there have been deaths. Unless you've a numbered offshore account or are a tech corporation with an Irish sweetheart, it is, as we all know, as inevitable as taxes. The settings are varied, the reasons diverse, but the net result the same.

Albert, my father's genial neighbour in Bath, who found me collapsed and naked when he dropped in with some sausages before taking control – he put me in some of Dad's bright lemon pyjamas and called for an ambulance – has left us. It was a crisp Saturday morning by the quarry outside Coleraine in Northern Ireland with no sign of impending danger, when the mechanical arm of the digger he was driving collapsed. Poor Albert was hurled through the cockpit and killed instantly. No warning, no sense of what was and now is, just a catatonic switch between alive and dead. Two young daughters and a loving family are devastated. This is the man I owe my life to who no longer is. He is now a 'was'. Where are those sausages?

Then there was David T, the rascal who took me to the Pump Room in Bath in a wheelchair without MOT: a chaotic journey that saw my returning on a wine list to give my poor buttocks some relief and David requiring a recuperative rest on my hospital bed. "It's my prostate," he told me a few years ago. "I've got cancer. But don't worry, I'm going to eat myself better with raw food. You should try it, raw chocolate, you can even clean your teeth with it."

"Just take the chuffing chemo you moron," I considerately replied. He was dead nine months later, a stiff frightened of becoming unable to get stiff. I loved his renegade spirit, hedonistic obsessions and crass mistakes, but couldn't love him for this. "You're committing suicide," I berated, but David T wouldn't listen. Thus one of my valued conspirators was gone.

If I'd had the chance I'd also have said goodbye to Peter Tapley who, with his wife Jane, provided a memorable supper party in the Bath hospital lobby – we had to bribe the cleaners to extend their fag break – complete with candelabra, roulade and Stinking Bishop cheese. He went to load up the car for a trip to his beloved Dartmouth and never came back. The heart attack was fatal, and the effect on Jane so cruel to witness at the funeral.

I must also mention Mike Stapleton, an old warrior in hotel finances, a roistering cantankerous guy with a heart of gold. Quick to berate me for overvaluing any hotel business he was nevertheless a good friend. Bless him, he 'got' my book to such an extent that he bought a copy for all of his family of 27, packed them into his suitcase (the books not the relatives) and cleared off one fine weekend to France to see them all – and promptly died. We had a breakfast in south London on the morning of his departure. I never saw him again but picture him in my mind every day. Cancer got him and the weight loss was profound before the passing.

Meanwhile the marvellous Mary, the woman who woke me most mornings at 6.30am, could do the work of three others with ease and discuss the finer points of the offside rule – and who somehow found time to nurse a son at home – is struggling. She has cancer and as I write is in a critical condition.

Talking of remarkable individuals who entered into my life through GBS, I really must mention Charles Delamain. He was the articulate, inspiring, young cavalier who'd returned to a high-velocity lifestyle after breaking his back diving into a pool at the age of 23, and wisely advised me to limit my response to enquiries about my health with the simple "Fine, thank you". Sadly the news is no brighter. One early April evening, when riding his moped around the perimeter of Buckingham Palace, he suffered an aneurysm and crashed into the garden wall: an instantly fatal accident.

Yet I can't think of Charles without flashing back to one savagely comical incident early in my recovery when he visited me in hospital. He was accompanied by his partner in crime, Madders, a man whose diverse career included a stint as auctioneer for India's IPL, selling off the world's finest cricketing talent to the highest bidding team. At the time the only emotional response available to my depleted body was to sweat: something I did profusely as Delamain leant down and whispered conspiratorially into my ear.

"I can't help but notice the lovely Suzi," he growled, smiling roguishly. "Like any woman she has needs, and this must be a tricky time for you both. If you'd like me to help out in that department, Robin, I'm only too happy to oblige; keep it in the family so to speak." My trickle of sweat morphed into a river, then a raging torrent. Yes, it was dark, but it was also funny. Seriously funny.

Unsurprisingly for someone whose life burned so brightly, Charles's funeral was standing room only: a dignified but fitting service. After the requisite hymns we left the church to his favourite song, the Doors' *Riders on the Storm*, the congregation *Pink Panther-ing* our way down the aisle to the familiar opening notes.

I apologise if this all seems to be getting a tad bleak. It really isn't meant to. As GBS taught me all those years ago, life, with its enormous lottery wins and catastrophes, isn't just something that happens to other people in the papers. Major events, the good, the bad, the ugly, affect all of us, and the last ten years have undoubtedly seen a balance of both: the ying and yang of existence.

While it simply isn't possible to keep up with most of the paths I crossed on the wards, I'm still friends with Sundance. He was always an unlikely ally, but with a friendship forged in adversity, we laughed at each other's misfortune and found a particularly British comfort in our mutual ineptitude. He still has MS, it goes without saying, but takes life as it comes with his children – those great markers of passing time – now 19 and 16.

And I'd like to approach closure with something positive. In fact, with something very positive that emerged directly from my experience with GBS. When I'd recovered my strength and faculties enough to venture out from the hospital, initially pushed in a wheelchair then using my Zimmer, I was astounded and frustrated by the difficulty – sometimes the outright impossibility – of access to many buildings. One particularly tricky entrance to a restaurant in Wimbledon, accompanied by Nigel, a friend visiting from Australia, springs to mind. Mostly for the ghastly obstacle course of negotiating my frame between its tables, but also for finding a chair of the right height that wouldn't slip on the floor as I sat down. Minor challenges compared to many others I was facing, of course, but nonetheless issues that can begin to be rectified with a little thought, effort and creativity.

So that's what I've done. The Bespoke Access Awards were launched at the House of Lords in spring 2016 with the aim of drawing attention to the value of good design in delivering hotel access for the disabled and those with learning difficulties. Already a success, it's now supported by many, including Channel 4, Hewi and Dyson, and has attracted superb entries from architects as far afield as Russia, Hong Kong, Germany and Canada, as well as the UK. The first winner, judged by a panel including a Paralympic gold medallist, Stirling Prize-winning architect and peer of the realm – I gave my two pence worth too – was announced in December of the same year. It's not the answer but it's a step, or perhaps shuffle, in the right direction. Something good out of something sad.

And I'd like to end on an uplifting personal note, after which I promise I really will put my pen down for the last time. In 2016 I was presented with the Outstanding Contribution gong at The Cateys, the hospitality industry's leading awards ceremony (and also presented with the same accolade at the Oxford Brookes Bacchus awards). It was a surreal experience to be congratulated by many of my heroes from the business including Robin Hutson – founder of the Hotel du Vin empire and the splendid collection of Pig properties – and Gordon Campbell Gray, creator of Beirut's iconic Le Gray Hotel and London's One Aldwych.

I'm sure it was a sympathy vote for an old cripple but I'll gladly accept it. I was in shock at hearing the news, and still am now: a state I'll happily endure after everything else I've been through in recent times. And with that final happy update I'll now take my leave for good.

- The End -

All proceeds from the sale of this book will be given to the GAIN Charity
to help fight the illness and raise funds for further research.

About the Author

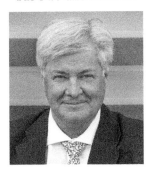

Robin Sheppard had always seemed like a lucky guy! Proud father of two sons in their late teens, Sam the elder (the musical one) and Charlie (the artistic one); still good friends with his first wife Georgina known always as George, and partnered by the effervescent and indomitable Suzanne known by all as Suzi, when his hitherto contented life took a different turn.

He had bounded through 50 years of an unfettered existence working in places that didn't feel like any factory or office you might know. A universe largely comprising five star hotels set in manicured gardens, with fine wines, fabulous foie gras, and outrageous flower arrangements, speckled with well-heeled customers in which the anticipation of their needs was paramount.

After growing up in Bath he had become a hotelier who delighted in operating some of the very best of Britain's hotels, winning 'hotel of the year' prizes along the way, before founding with some like-minded chums their own specialist hotel-operating group. Ending up in London he presided over an empire of a dozen or so glamorous hotels which featured architecture of the Grade 1 variety, decadent décor, period fixtures in Capability Brown parkland surroundings, and food of the highest standard. His was an untroubled workplace.

Taking time out along the way to invent the truly iconic, deep-blue, skittle-shaped, Ty-Nant mineral water business and then a niche adult soft drinks business, he became an entrepreneur without ever knowing it and a role model for many a novice hotel student along the way.

Then things changed.